"The neglected subject in the Black community is now an open, honest book. In this instructive volume, 'pause' means 'power,' where the Second Half becomes the Better Half."

> —Dr. Gwendolyn Goldsby Grant, *Essence* columnist and author of *The Best Kind of Loving*

"This book is right on time! Do yourself and the African heritage women you care about a favor—get a copy for each one to use as they journey through perimenopause and menopause."

> —Dr. Beverly Yates, author of *Heart Health for Black Women*

"A groundbreaking book. *The Black Woman's Guide to Menopause* speaks directly to Black women, giving them the information they need to do menopause with an attitude."

> —Carolle Jean-Murat, M.D., author of *Menopause Made Easy*

"Kudos to Brown and Levy for an upbeat book that prescribes celebration, affirmation, spiritual exploration, and education with a dash of sassy attitude as medicine to ease our spirits through one of life's most challenging transitions."

> —Stephanie Rose Bird, *Sage Woman* magazine columnist

"Carolyn Scott Brown is lyrical in the exploration of the psychological and biological manifestations of menopause."

> —Gale Madyun, founder/president of local Older Women's League chapter

The Black Woman's Guide to Menopause

Doing Menopause with Heart and Soul

Carolyn Scott Brown

with Barbara S. Levy, M.D.

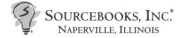

SOURCEBOOKS, INC.®
NAPERVILLE, ILLINOIS

Published by Sourcebooks, Inc.
P.O. Box 4410, Naperville, Illinois 60567-4410
(630) 961-3900
FAX: (630) 961-2168
www.sourcebooks.com

Library of Congress Cataloging-in-Publication Data

Scott Brown, Carolyn.
  The Black woman's guide to menopause / by Carolyn Scott Brown, with Barbara S. Levy.
      p. ; cm.
  Includes bibliographical references.
  ISBN 1-57071-933-0 (alk. paper)
  1. Menopause—Popular works. 2. African American women—Health and hygiene—Popular works.
  [DNLM: 1. Menopause—Popular Works. 2. Blacks—Popular Works. 3. Women's Health—Popular Works. WP 580 S425b 2003] I. Title.
RG186.S414 2003
618.1'75—dc21

                         2003005074

Printed and bound in the United States of America
BG 10 9 8 7 6 5 4 3 2 1

This book is dedicated to my mom, Alonza, and
my friend Jewell, two women I loved dearly.
They lived their lives with grace, wisdom,
and compassion for others.

Acknowledgments

Carolyn Scott Brown:

I'd like to thank my mom for being such a rock in my life and for always sharing her menopausal journey. Thanks to my husband Lester for his tenderness, positive energy, and emotional support. I appreciate my sister LaVerne for being in my corner and helping me with each stage of researching and writing this book. Thanks to Aunt Marie, Ruby, Shirlene, Aunt Olivia, Joan, Charlye, and Pat and all the awesome women in my family for sharing their stories.

Special thanks to our agent Felicia Eth for believing in our message from the beginning. We appreciate our editors Hillel Black and Laura Kuhn for their expertise in working on the manuscript. Thanks to Molly Strasser and all the great people at Sourcebooks.

My sister friends have been invaluable to this project because of their willingness to share their thoughts and feelings about perimenopause and menopause. I am grateful to Branice, Pauline, Bits, Jessie, Natilyn, Jackie, Floretta, Fern, Carolyn, Dolores, Fran, Linda, Bridgette, Judith, June, Deborah, and Darlene.

I am deeply grateful to Dr. Gwendolyn Goldsby Grant, Dr. Carolle Jean-Murat, Dr. Beverly Yates, and Dr. Shawne Bryant for their support.

BARBARA LEVY:

I'd like to thank my wonderful patients who teach me and help me learn every day by sharing their lives and their stories.

Table of Contents

Introduction

We, the Black women who are constantly being told how strong and powerful we are, experience times in our lives when we feel overwhelmed and discouraged about what the future holds. We want to live more authentic lives and ground ourselves in a journey that reaffirms our spirit, a spirit that makes the grand dames of our past proud. But sometimes we are too involved in the complexity of our lives to focus on how to achieve that goal. What would Sojourner Truth or Harriet Tubman have to say about the way we lead our lives? I ask myself if they feel we are carrying the torch in a manner worthy of the good fight they fought.

I wrote this book for African-American women who, like me, are trying to find a way to age gracefully and achieve a new kind of success at midlife. There seems to be a feeling among us that we don't have the time or the patience to cope with perimenopause and menopause. Sadly, these feelings will result in our wasting too much time before we grasp the main lessons to be learned at midlife, and we will delay the positive benefits gained from doing menopause with a new attitude. Taking the time to discover a new path through menopause takes courage, forethought, and insight. We must be prepared to dig deep inside to master this transition.

There are many things I wish someone had told me about this journey before I started my transition so that I could have found my way in a more conscious manner. Now I want to take you on this journey and share with you the lessons I learned. A successful voyage involves nurturing the mind, body, and spirit, tasks we African-American women often ignore. I discovered there are eight steps to master before we can truly celebrate menopause. Before we get started, I am here to tell you that perimenopause and menopause serve as a wake-up call reminding us that taking care of ourselves has to be faced and that we can't afford to ignore the connection between mind and body. Using the power of our minds to reframe our thoughts and beliefs about menopause is the solution to healing our bodies.

Knowledge is power, and there is nothing more powerful than learning to use our minds to help us improve our health at midlife. Being Black and female in America carries with it many challenges and unique stresses, but the real challenge for us African-American women is not coping with the biological symptoms like hot flashes and vaginal dryness, it is resolving the psychological baggage we drag along with us into this amazing transitional period. Mastery of this "stuff" can be a gateway into a more authentic existence because the roles we have been playing that don't resonate with our inner beings should be adjusted and discarded at this juncture. We must complete the spiritual and mind/body work necessary to take us within. The strategies and menopause action plans I share with you for celebrating the Second Half of Life are defined as mind/body medicine, strategies that beckon us to get in touch, in tune, renewed, empowered, jazzed, or whatever you want to call it. A lot of time and energy is not required to master these techniques, but a commitment to living consciously and increasing our awareness of what makes us happy is important.

Menopause, I am convinced, has a lot to do with building personal power and aligning cognitive and emotional patterns so that we respond appropriately to the challenges and circumstances we encounter during midlife. Effectively managing our mental, emotional, and physical symptoms is no easy task, but the end result of moving to a state of rebirth and renewal is worth it.

Moving toward an alpha state where we celebrate our African heritage and our experience of this phase is the goal. It is a state where our symptoms are managed superbly, our mental and emotional needs are met, and we are nourishing our minds and bodies with the style and grace that is the trademark of proud African-American women.

Moving away from a beta state where we are bogged down with biological symptoms, easily stressed, and out of sync with our inner feelings is the direction we want to go. Positive, forward movement is necessary, as we can't re-create the past and we can't stand still, because menopause is the stepping stone to a more meaningful phase of life.

We must become more willing to change and develop our thinking skills to a point where we approach this transition with childlike wonder and open-mindedness. Sisters, it is time for us to evolve to another level of existence filled with mindfulness and purpose, a purpose tied to being more than the challenges we face.

We have interpreted the studies, books, and available information about this passage, which is so different from what our mothers experienced. The eight steps are based on the experiences of the hundreds of Black women we have talked to, counseled, and treated. They came to us with their questions, fears, and thoughts about how this journey would impact their lives. Step two on the biological factors and medical information related to menopause, step four on mood disorders, and step six on complementary medicine and wellness are each covered in two chapters.

I am on a mission to start a movement for African-American women on how to change our transition by intent and to do it with heart and soul. I conceived of and wrote this book with Dr. Barbara Levy because she shared every step of this journey with me. She extended herself above and beyond what I expected. We spent many hours just talking about my life, my health, her life, the roles of Black women and white women, and what we each bring to midlife. Many people have asked why I am writing a book for Black women with a white doctor as my coauthor. I tell them she is instrumental in my story, and our collaboration on my healing is very much on point.

Chapter 1 reminds us that we can't afford to ignore the mind-body connection. It's time to use our minds to develop a new perspective, new thoughts, and new attitudes about menopause. We must adopt new beliefs about what is possible for us at midlife.

Chapters 2 and 3 describe how to explore our options and get educated about menopause. First, we explore the research and latest information about the biological changes that take place and then we teach women strategies for coping with the medical conditions that Black women are prone to develop. The "how tos" of how to prevent heart disease, diabetes, breast cancer, obesity, and osteoporosis are covered with simple tips and recommendations.

Chapter 4 discusses the benefits of establishing a meaningful partnership with a primary caregiver and reviews the role each of us must play in becoming accountable for our health care. The importance of Black women learning to become proactive in their journey is reviewed. I ask you questions like, Why do we mistrust the medical establishment? How can we get over it and move on? What does it take for us stop neglecting our own care?

Chapters 5 and 6 explore the topic of mood disorders, starting with a review of the latest information on mood disorders, depression, and "the blues." In chapter 5, we help you determine where you are on the continuum from bad moods to clinical depression. New information makes it clear that menopause does not cause depression, but learning how to manage stress, handle our anger, and get our priorities in order are the keys to mastering mood disorders. Some of us may need medical help, depending on the type of baggage we carry into this transition. Girlfriends, we know we have issues that are particular to our situations and our tendency to repress our feelings, and chapter 6 reveals strategies for dealing with these feelings. Sisters, we must learn to get our anger in check. Black women are angry about a multitude of things, some of it justified and some of it misguided, but regardless of the cause, we have to shake it off so we can get well.

In chapter 7, we take a look at how African-American women are often stereotyped as "sexy" and "too hot to handle." These stereotypes are a source of ethnic pride and a symbol of our earthy sensuality, but they also put us in a box that dictates how we are expected to behave. Possibly we are allowing ourselves to play roles that are not relevant or that feed into negative stereotypes that impede our growth and development. Almost every sister I talk to wants to know how perimenopause and menopause will impact her sexuality. Some of us want to know but are afraid to discuss it. It's time to face all the fears and myths about sex after fifty. We encourage you to talk with your partner and to work on maintaining your sexuality whether or not you have a partner.

Chapters 8 and 9 trace our cultural heritage as it relates to complementary healing and reviews the latest information on wellness behavior, nutrition, and so-called "alternative medicine." We also encourage you to design your own Personal Health Success Plan and find an accountability partner to help you achieve your goals.

Chapter 10 talks about the emotional benefits of sharing this journey with your "sister friends," other Black women who can relate to what your life is like. I also discuss how to start a culturally appropriate menopause group. While reaching out to our sisters, let's commit to eliminating the barriers to true sisterhood and get rid of historical feelings that lead us to mistreat other Black women because of their skin tone, social status, and level of education. The way we treat or mistreat our own is related to how we treat ourselves. These biases are not worthy of us. We all have to deal with the consequences of living in a land where our ancestors were enslaved. There is value in maintaining and enhancing our relationships with women from other ethnic groups during menopause. Some of what we experience is comparable. Our relationships with our white female friends are valuable and we can learn valuable lessons from them all. Some of our challenges are quite similar.

Becoming a full leader in your own life is the message in chapter 11. Guide your life based on principles and values that help you achieve your purpose and vision. Live your life with courage and foresight and take risks that move you toward your dreams after effectively managing your physical and emotional symptoms.

Join us on this journey to mastering the Second Half of Life!

Celebrate the Second Half of Life

WHAT IS MENOPAUSE AND WHAT DO AFRICAN-AMERICAN WOMEN THINK ABOUT IT?

Menopause is the time after a woman experiences her last menstrual period along with changes throughout her body as a result of reduced estrogen in the body. For African-American women, these changes can be aggravated by belief systems and behavior patterns based on our need to see ourselves as invincible. The self-imposed burden of being all things to all people is another factor that influences our attitudes about midlife transition. Psychologically, menopause is a time when we are challenged to reevaluate our lives and our plans for what we want to accomplish in the next thirty or possibly forty years.

It's interesting to note how our thoughts, attitudes, and expectations impact our transition. For women like us, the first step in changing our attitudes about menopause involves understanding that experiencing menopause successfully is a mind game. We need to change our minds about this passage. We must make our emotional, mental, and spiritual health a higher priority. If you are anything like me, maybe you don't think you have been neglecting your own self-care.

Maybe you haven't had time to think about the "the change," as our mothers called it. I hadn't thought a lot about it, but when faced with the passage,

I had anticipated that I would be more enlightened. I was shocked to find myself feeling fearful and anxious about being perceived as old. When I became aware of dreading this passage, it hit me like a ton of bricks. I shocked myself. You must understand that worrying about getting old has never been a problem for me. Although I have girlfriends who are always obsessing about their next birthdays, I never understood where they were coming from until my own negative feelings about aging came to the surface. I always said that as long as I kept getting better and achieving my goals, I didn't have time to think about aging. But entering menopause abruptly at age forty-four got my attention. I began to focus on the negative perceptions of others as well as the nature of my own conditioning. My thought was, "I'm not ready to deal with this aging thing." But never one to run from a challenge, I decided that designing a new approach was in order.

I know cultural conditioning plays a strong role in our perceptions of menopause and aging. I have always been interested in anthropology and I can truly say I have always been fascinated by the impact culture has on our behavior. Actually, when I was younger, I wanted to be the African-American Margaret Mead, so exploring the role that cultural conditioning plays in determining our behavior at midlife comes naturally to me. As you are well aware, our cultural conditioning as African-American women is to be strong and invincible, but there is also a need to be perceived as feminine and desirable.

This calls for a dichotomy in the way we live our lives because we have to be strong and powerful women who must also maintain a certain aura of feminine mystique. It has been my experience that Black men have trouble coping with us when they perceive us as being too assertive, even though they like to brag about how "bodacious" and "outrageous" we can be. It's a catch-22. The men in my life have always said they loved my independent nature, but there have been times when I know they were threatened by it.

Also, I didn't do a good job of letting them know when I needed emotional support. Asking for help is something I don't do well. Maybe you can relate to that. Well, now we have an opportunity to let our men see our vulnerability and to ask the brothers to help us make the transition. As we come to grips with our own thoughts and feelings, we must address theirs as well. All this work must be done in a manner that facilitates our celebration of the Second Half of Life.

Our African-American ancestors revered older women. It is part of our culture to value older women as powerful, but the degree to which you and I have internalized Western beliefs that devalue women is a measure of how far we have moved away from our African heritage. It doesn't help that we live in a society where beauty is always tied to being young. I have always felt comfortable with my level of attractiveness and somehow assumed it wouldn't change with age. The older women in my family are still beautiful and are living meaningful lives. My perception of them has always been that they are happy and feel comfortable in their skin. Now I wonder if they felt diminished during menopause, or if they ever felt the need to rebel.

BECOMING A MENOPAUSE REBEL

We cope with discrimination on two fronts and we know what it feels like to be the underdog. Challenging the beliefs and expectations of others comes easily to us. Since I have rebelled against every feminine role that didn't suit me, changing the way I perceived menopause was a logical step for me. My new attitude has helped me eliminate feelings of shame about what is basically a natural stage of development. I have rejected sexism and racism and now I reject ageism. So can you.

This book will help you review, explore, and adjust your attitudes about menopause, aging, and the Second Half of Life. We have overcome many ethnic- and gender-related stereotypes as our tremendous achievements have begun to be recognized, but you and I as African-American women in midlife now have age-related stereotypes to overcome. People like to categorize us, when in reality we don't fit any single mold, and every day we are reinventing ourselves as we face new challenges. We are treading new ground as the first generation of Black "baby boomers" with the opportunity to really celebrate menopause, so it makes sense for all of us to redirect our energy toward seeing this passage as a gateway to a new beginning.

What's Attitude Got To Do With It?

You might be unclear about what attitude has to do with it. Research studies show that attitudes and beliefs about menopause are culturally defined. If you have any doubts about the importance of attitudes, take a look at the research on cultural differences in how menopause is experienced. In cultures where older women are highly respected, hot flashes and other typically Western symptoms are nonexistent. Japanese and Native American cultures are examples of cultures that value older women. As a result, this perception has traditionally caused women in these cultures to experience less trauma about aging. Many of us women of color have moved away from traditional beliefs, so our feelings about aging have changed accordingly.

Often, we are unaware of all of our cultural beliefs. As we give you a blueprint for examining this issue, and as you explore ways to help determine whether you are carrying any negative attitudes about this passage, I hope you will be challenged, as I was, to substitute new attitudes and beliefs about the way you approach your menopause.

Because negative feelings about aging chipped away at my feelings about my desirability, it initially made me more vulnerable to the negative perceptions of others. Allowing myself to focus on losses during menopause led me to begin seeing myself as "less than." In order to keep others from devaluing me, I had to place a higher value on myself at this juncture and recapture my sense of self. I decided to develop a new culturally sensitive midlife identity. Many of my beliefs were so ingrained that I didn't realize how they influenced my behavior until I faced my fears and changed my conditioning. I used cognitive menopause strategies like visualization, affirmation, and mentoring, which I have used to help African-American women control stress and make positive changes in their lives. I sought out strong, vibrant African-American female role models who have successfully conquered this transition with grace and power. All of these strategies will be shared in this book.

How we deal with and come through menopause will set us up to have a wonderful Second Half of Life because menopause is a rite of passage to a better future if we develop positive attitudes. Attitudes are so significant because our attitude determines the way we view things. When we have a positive attitude toward a situation, circumstance, or passage, we expect positive things to happen and lean toward them with a positive expectancy. When we have a negative attitude, we have a negative expectancy and lean away from the situation, event, or passage with dread. I worked on adjusting my attitude until I found myself leaning toward menopause and doing it with a new attitude.

For me it means:
- I eliminated any sense of shame about my experience.
- I demanded answers and refused to let anyone devalue me.
- I let go of old attitudes and stereotypes that are no longer relevant.
- I continued to talk about my experiences to increase awareness and break down the barriers imposed by society.
- I educated myself. I educated others. I made my cultural conditioning work for me.

What can you do?

+ Rebel against that garbage that makes you afraid.
+ Reject any put-downs or patronizing attitudes from others.
+ Don't be a victim to midlife, be a winner.

WHAT HAVE WE AFRICAN-AMERICAN WOMEN HEARD ABOUT MENOPAUSE?

When asked what they have heard about menopause, African-American women repeated the following statements. Check them out and see if you can relate to them:

+ Menopause is the beginning of old age.
+ Our femininity and desirability will diminish during menopause.
+ Weight gain is automatic.
+ Hot flashes can't be controlled.
+ Mood swings are a trip.
+ You fall apart and can't take care of your business.
+ It messes with your life.
+ Menopause is the end.
+ Your husband starts to see you as an old broad.
+ Your feelings are easily hurt.
+ You become hard to get along with.
+ Your testosterone increases and you become more aggressive.
+ Your life is over.
+ It's not so bad. My mom was OK with it.

Looking at these myths will help you pinpoint how you feel about this transition.

WHAT DOES MENOPAUSE FEEL LIKE?

There's a wealth of information about menopausal symptoms, but when I began my journey, I couldn't find enough information describing how menopause feels. As Black women, we are closely tied to our inner voices, intuition, and gut-level reactions to circumstances. Our feelings and perceptions of danger have saved our lives, and we are masters at gauging the threat in any situation. We need to understand how things will feel. It was upsetting to me to find that the current books barely addressed cultural and ethnic differences in the way menopause is experienced. Much of the information available on menopause was confusing and irrelevant to me as an African-American woman. Maybe what happens physiologically is the same for all women, but what we bring to these hormonal and bodily changes and how we respond to what our bodies are going through has everything to do with who we are as African-American women.

As I encouraged African-American women to talk about menopause and perimenopause, I received a variety of responses. Some were reluctant to discuss it with me. Others were embarrassed to hear me speaking openly about something that they feel is very private, secretive, and perhaps shameful. Still others said that because it is a natural phase of life, they didn't expect to have any problems. That had been my sentiment exactly, but life has a way of testing us. Initially, I failed the "midlife challenge test" because I wasn't in touch with my true feelings.

Unfortunately, in the past, African-American women who were experiencing difficulty during menopause did not feel comfortable discussing their feelings and therefore were not able to share their experiences. It is still something of a taboo today. If they had been encouraged to talk to other women, they would have learned that menopause is a unique experience for each of us. The following reflects some of their general comments about menopause:

During menopause, I lost my ability to experience joy in life and everyone irritated me—my husband, children, and coworkers. When I could no longer ignore how bad I was feeling, I finally talked to my doctor, who suggested that I could be in menopause. Immediately, I felt better because I was beginning to think that I was going crazy.

My menopause was so easy. I flashed and had insomnia for a couple of months and then boom, my cycle just stopped. I was so happy to be finished with my period that I ignored the other changes.

One day I found myself sweating while everyone else was apparently comfortable. Sweat was running down my face and back. It was very embarrassing. I didn't want to believe that I was having a hot flash until this happened several times in one day.

I got real depressed, but I thought it was because my daughter went away to college. But finally, I realized that it was more than that. I started putting things together and it became obvious that I was in menopause.

I heard my mother and grandmother say their level of sexual activity and interest diminished after menopause. I don't feel that way. I feel my life really became my own after menopause. My desire for sex is stronger than ever. My husband says I need to give it a rest.

Menopause is a life transition and since our lifespan is getting longer, get used to menopause.

Girl, I'm not ready to start thinking about getting that old. I don't talk about it and none of my friends are talking about it.

CHECKING OUT MY REALITY

I thought about my mother's menopause and realized that she didn't talk much about her psychological response to the "change." I developed more of a preoccupation with things like gray hair, wrinkles, and middle-age spread. I was more conscious of my gray hairs and checking for wrinkles even when I knew that I barely had any. I had to take time and really think about what was so threatening about reaching menopause. Fortunately, there was a positive outcome to doing some soul-searching.

This transition motivated me to begin to think about being the best *me*. I realized I didn't want to waste any more time talking about my goals. I made the time to do some of the things I had been postponing, such as writing a book, learning a new language, taking golf lessons, reestablishing contacts with old girlfriends, and learning to draw.

African-American women are so invested in being indomitable and responding fast without thinking. But the Second Half of Life demands that we slow down, look within, and then relaunch ourselves with a new focus on nurturing the self. Menopause will get our attention. It's hard to ignore the biological changes, but we may attempt to ignore the psychological aspects because we are so good at compartmentalizing our feelings.

For many Black women, menopause is a time when we feel more in touch with our bodies. We begin to appreciate the essence of who we are inside, perhaps allowing our softer side to emerge. Along with our enhanced feelings of confidence, we also feel a sense of glory and increased sensuality. For me, it's like I blossomed into a warmer, more accepting alter ego.

I also learned to detach myself from some of my self-imposed pressures and take the time to feel really good while I contemplated what I wanted to do differently in the next phase of my life. This frame of mind did not come easily. I struggled with my approach for a while. Once I faced the fact that my symptoms were real, I gave up on my attempt to use old defense mechanisms. You know what I'm talking about! I had to get real, face my fears, and see this journey as a positive, self-affirming opportunity.

Many women report more energy, zest, excitement, and focus during menopause. It's a time of great change, but also a time of great inner contentment. Although there are times when you may feel anxious because of lack of control, a part of you knows you can handle it.

Take advice from my cousin Ruby:

> *I am 50 and proud of it. I look better and feel better about myself. I'm dating a much younger man. He chose me because I was not looking. I wouldn't know if I was in menopause. I do know that I did my job. I raised my two kids and paid for their education. I don't look to anybody to make me happy. Being older is a blessing. All the younger women at work look to me for advice. Send me one of those Do Menopause with an Attitude T-shirts and I'll be happy to wear it.*

In order to appreciate menopause from this life-affirming point of view, several things need to happen.

You must have the right caregiver, someone who cares about you and helps you relax enough to really admit when you need help. You also need someone who encourages you to participate in your healing. My initial contacts with Dr. Barbara Levy were productive and informative. I left our first few appointments with the feeling that I could master midlife issues with her assistance.

You need to allow yourself to feel capable of being an active partner in planning and designing your treatment plan. It's really about accountability. We always think we can overcome anything, which is true, but the *how* is another matter. Our methods for overcoming and fighting back may not be effective in the Second Half of Life because a gentler approach is required. Midlife is a good time to write in a journal, keep a calendar of your flashes, moods, sleep patterns, diet, exercise routines, and any changes that occur. You have to face the reality of what's happening to you. Writing things down helps make them real.

When I started keeping a menopause journal, I realized I was "flashing," unable to concentrate, and moody. For months after my surgery, I tried to avoid dealing with these symptoms. As I said before, I was in denial big-time. Once I went back to Dr. Levy and worked closely with her in a successful partnership, we put together the right combination of treatment modalities and I began to take the time to figure out what I needed and how to take care of myself.

You must give up the role of being in charge and totally in control. Maintaining control is a big thing for us. We don't want anyone to tell us what to do, even when it is appropriate. We have a sense of power honed to sharpness by coping with and fighting centuries of racism and sexism. We hide our feelings from most people except our trusted girlfriends. Unfortunately, our girlfriends tend to have the same warrior mentality and may not be able to tell us when it's time to slow down and tune in to what we need to do for our bodies and spirits. Although your sense of being in control will come back, there is a time during the beginning of menopause when you have to let your body be in charge. We have to take note of how wise the body is as it moves you toward the next stage of development. "Your body will let you know what it needs," Dr. Levy constantly reminds me.

I found myself being driven to do things differently. It was as if my body knew it needed more fresh foods and grains. It was hard for me to be careless about what I ate. I didn't crave traditional high-fat soul food. I was used to drinking at least eighty ounces of water each day, but I actually began to crave more water. I also felt the need to be more focused on my moods and my spiritual journey. There were days when I felt out of control.

I learned to roll with the flow. I wrote letters to Dr. Levy clearly describing my experiences and offered suggestions about what I thought I needed. Sometimes I was way off-base, but at least I was actively involved in getting myself well. Focusing on every aspect of my health became my number one priority. My mom and my sister LaVerne were very nurturing during this time and we talked almost daily during the first chaotic year of my menopause.

Understand that menopause is a process. It is not a point of arrival. It is a passage to a new stage or space where your body, mind, and spirit are renewed and blossom like the beginning of springtime. There's a feeling of a new awakening, but at the same time you shed part of your old self and all the baggage that goes with it.

I thought about drawing on all the strengths of my ancestors and how Black women have always been pathfinders. It is part of our heritage to know when it is time to do something different. My friend Jean says, "Girl, I just go with the flow. Little things don't bug me these days. I do what I think is right and let the chips fall where they may. I don't have time to do everything right."

Don't let other people tell you things that cause you to doubt your feelings. I knew that something strange was going on with me, but when I tried to talk to some of my friends, they couldn't relate. They didn't want to get into it because they wanted to postpone thinking about menopause.

We have devised a plan that encompasses new attitudes about aging. It involves spending more time in the Second Half of Life being true to ourselves and our passion for living an extraordinary and fulfilling lives. What does that mean to you? Once you answer that question, you will be on the road to an interesting menopause journey. For me, it meant taking the time to reevaluate how I spend my time and making sure I am using my creative gifts to do work that truly makes me happy. I also decided I didn't want to run and hide from middle age. Finally, my perception of what's important in life has changed. My future growth and development is tied to how well I handle the challenges of the Second Half of Life and it has become important to me to be honest with myself about the amount of time I have been spending trying to please others. Maybe you can relate to that.

A Baby Boomer Turns Fifty Every Seven Minutes

Some of us African-American boomers are the first generation in our families to enjoy a comfortable lifestyle. We are living a life that our mothers never even dreamed of. Like all boomers, we tend to question all the old myths at each stage of development and it is necessary to question the status quo with menopause so we can take it out of the closet. Because there is so much information available to us about menopause, it is easier to look at all the options available before making treatment decisions. But we have no footsteps to follow in the psychological realm during this phase because no one has forged this particular path before. We are the pioneers of a new way of doing menopause where the psychological and spiritual aspects are valued as much as the biological. We have options about how we redefine the aging process for African-American women after the age of forty. How we are coping with the pressure of having to prove ourselves over and over again is a good question to answer at midlife.

How are we coping with the way the world perceives us? We are successful in many ways, but at what cost to our psychological and spiritual health? I'm sure you and I can easily count the status symbols we have accrued as a group of women. We are triumphing every day as we get more education, nontraditional jobs, start our own businesses, or move up the corporate ladder and raise our families in environments that offer them tremendous opportunities. But we are angry because we have to be twice as good at everything. I haven't always handled that anger well, and maybe you haven't either. As we are fond of saying, "Black women have issues," and these issues need to be addressed in midlife so our journey can be one of self-actualization.

Many of us have reached a level of economic freedom that allows us to support ourselves without being financially dependent on anyone. We have more alternatives tied to deciding who we are and what we are capable of achieving. This freedom creates a dilemma because sometimes the more success we achieve, the more alienated we begin to feel from our roots and our community. Some of us are the first generation of our families to attend college or have jobs that count for more than "trading time for money." Learning how to live in harmony with our strong need to succeed and still maintain strong cultural ties is a big job, but many of us are quite successful at merging the two worlds. We learn to live with a lot of stress that may manifest itself in different ways during menopause. We have used up most of our inner reserves before entering this phase of life. Our negative attitudes about menopause may be related to our feelings that our plates are already too full.

Life Lesson

Often we function in a working world that is totally different from the environment we live in, and we deal with many situations that are not culturally affirming. We find moving back and forth between both worlds takes skill and an awareness of the tremendous value of our cultural ties. I have always maintained my bond with my family and my old community. Whenever I return to Detroit for visits, I am reminded of my past and the valuable lessons I learned there. More than 70 percent of my high-school class attended college. This was a first for my high school. Many of my friends remained in Michigan and are achieving their goals; some attended college elsewhere and returned home within a few years. In my family, I was the first one who ventured farther away, but I have committed to staying "real" because being authentic is one of my core values. My philosophy is serving me well during the Second Half of Life. I am open and free about my experiences and what has happened to me during this journey. Remembering where I came from helps me use strengths gained from my environment, my community, and my extended family.

Only after coming to grips with our expectations and beliefs about who we are at this important turning point will we be able to break down our mental barriers to being more fulfilled at midlife.

Answer the following questions as you begin to check out your beliefs about menopause.

- What are your assumptions about menopause?
- How did you develop these assumptions?
- What do you expect menopause to be like?
- What does our culture tell us about aging?
- Are you ready for this?
- Whose beliefs have you adopted?
- What do you say to yourself about perimenopause/menopause?
- Who is your beacon in midlife?

Some Black women view menopause as a time to be free and start a wonderful new stage of life without the problems associated with a monthly cycle, PMS, cramps, and other reproductive problems. Others appear to be defensive about perimenopause and menopause and see this transition as the beginning of old age. They focus on perceived losses and are locked into old thought patterns, where women are primarily valued according to youthful standards of beauty and are defined by their appearances.

Which category matches your picture?

- Do you want to be fearful or fearless?

- Do you want to be seen as big and strong or small and weak?
- Do you want to run toward the next phase of your life or run away from it?

If we change the way we think, we will change the way we act!

- What steps will you take to prepare yourself for this major turning point in your life?
- Do you feel capable of taking a positive approach to this phase of your life?
- What is the biggest attitudinal obstacle you have to overcome?

THE ROLE OF CONDITIONING IN MENOPAUSE

In order to start changing our attitudes, beliefs, and assumptions, we have to come to grips with how we have been conditioned about menopause. Simply, conditioning means getting used to things. We are conditioned to see things in a certain way based on our past experiences and perceptions of life events. When we do things, see things, and hear things over and over, we begin to believe that what we are hearing, seeing, or believing is the truth. We build a scotoma, or "blind spot," to the real truth because we only see what we are used to seeing or what we expect to see.

Cultural conditioning is a process whereby we develop culturally biased assumptions and beliefs about the world. These beliefs determine our behavior. The way we perceive menopause is based on what our culture has taught us to believe about this transition. We are also influenced and conditioned by the larger culture of the world we live in. Our circle of influence starts with our families, neighborhood, and community, but by the time we are adults we have been influenced by the wider culture of this country through socialization and through the media.

Think back over your life. What have you been used to hearing about menopause?

"POSSIBILITY THINKING" IS AN ATTITUDE

Seeing exciting possibilities in our future at midlife is an attitude. We can adopt this attitude after increasing our understanding about how beliefs, attitudes, and expectations affect our perception of the truth. We act in accordance to the truth as we know it or believe it to be. Our perception of midlife transition is a powerful determinant of what we will expect. Some of us are perceptive enough to already face this transition without fear. My hat is off to you because the truth or reality of our experiences will correspond with our beliefs. Once we are aware of our ingrained beliefs and thought patterns, we can change them by changing our beliefs about what's possible for us at this time in our lives.

Ask yourself what's possible for you at this point in your life. What's holding you back or interfering with your ability to see new opportunities? How can possibility thinking change the way you handle your menopause?

Remember, the only limits on your potential are self-imposed by your thinking. Once you "lock on" to seeing your Second Half of Life as a time of unique possibilities, you will "lock out" negative thoughts and begin to see areas where you can grow and blossom.

To look at perimenopause/menopause differently, think about the following:

♦ It is a spiritual journey, a time to look inward.
♦ It is a time to get your priorities in order and to take the time to enjoy life while achieving your greatest accomplishments in all areas of your life.
♦ It is a time to do the things you have been postponing. It's now or never.
♦ It is a time to take stock of your life and make sure you are living according to your own rules.

♦ It is a time to make pleasing yourself just as important as pleasing others.

STEREOTYPES

Our conditioning has been influenced by stereotypes. Stereotypes are highly simplified opinions or beliefs about a group of people. These beliefs are automatically applied to everyone in that group without regard for individual differences. There are many negative stereotypes about women in menopause that we have all been exposed to over the years. We often think in terms of stereotypes without realizing it. The question is how stereotypes about menopause have impacted our attitudes about this transition. As Black women, we must redefine this passage for each other.

NOTES ABOUT STEREOTYPES

Why do people stereotype?

♦ To relieve anxiety in situations outside of their cultural comfort zones
♦ To make things predictable
♦ To help them deal with the fear of the unknown

Why are stereotypes so inaccurate?

♦ They are based on myths
♦ They do not take all factors and conditions into account
♦ They do not allow for individual differences based on education, socioeconomic status, motivation, etc.

Why are stereotypes dangerous?

♦ They interfere with our ability to see our potential
♦ They allow people to categorize others and avoid seeing them as they really are

♦ They can become self-fulfilling prophecies
♦ They are based on distorted thinking

Take time to think about the way African-American menopausal women are stereotyped. Take time to think about how you, as an African-American woman, have stereotyped menopause in your thinking. Eliminate negative conditioning by substituting positive thoughts and pictures about peri-menopause and menopause.

The following Menopause Mission Statement is a blueprint for our new approach. Read it. Think about it. Change it if you are so inclined, but use it to help you change your perspective about this journey

AFRICAN-AMERICAN WOMEN IN PERIMENOPAUSE/MENOPAUSE MISSION STATEMENT

We commit ourselves to maintaining our joy in life, to celebrate and glorify this most important rite of passage. We commit ourselves to building attitudes that are conducive to renewal, empowerment, and self-actualization for the next thirty or forty years. We also commit to learning about how our cultural conditioning impacts our behavior during menopause. We focus on eliminating old preconceptions and mis-judgments about the Second Half of Life for women of color.

Before reading farther, take a few moments and design a Menopause Mission Statement for yourself. Use the questions listed below to guide you.

Reflective questions
♦ How do you want the next thirty years of your life to unfold?
♦ What aspects of your life do you want to improve?
♦ What will be your legacy?

Do likewise with the Perimenopause/Menopause Bill of Rights. Use it as your personal proclamation.

PERIMENOPAUSE/MENOPAUSE BILL OF RIGHTS

◆ As beautiful Black women transitioning into perimenopause/menopause, we are healthy, happy, and enjoy a high-quality lifestyle.

◆ We are entitled to the best health care at midlife.

◆ We command respect from our spouses, partners, children, friends, and coworkers.

◆ We seek health-care providers who listen and value every aspect of our experiences and our cultural perspective on aging.

◆ We recognize the value of a positive and supportive network of friends and family.

◆ We reject ridicule, put-downs, and discrimination.

◆ We are kind to ourselves.

◆ We reach out to other women and support them on their journeys.

◆ We learn from our African-American ancestors and our cultural traditions.

◆ We realize we are in control of our attitudes, expectations, and beliefs.

THINGS TO THINK ABOUT

We tend to be very efficacious about our ability to control our lives, but these feelings can be threatened by the upheavals brought about by adjusting to menopause and perimenopause. The rest of this chapter will help you develop new cognitive menopause strategies like visualizing an exciting transition, affirming a sense of rejuvenation, and seeing change as an opportunity. Seek out strong, vibrant African-American female role models who have successfully conquered this transition with grace and power.

It's well-known that Native American cultures tend to view older women as wise and give them valued roles in the community. This contributes to a sense of perceiving menopause and aging as a positive part of the life cycle. We need to revisit that type of traditional cultural wisdom, which used to be more widely accepted in our own culture.

African-American women in menopause don't worry as much about appearing old because our skin pigmentation delays wrinkling and we don't usually look our age until about age seventy. This factor helps soften the blow a little. African-American women are often seen as powerful matriarchs, which contributes to our sense of being in control of our lives. But life is a paradox. On one hand we feel perennially young, but on the other hand we are looking at turning fifty soon—and reaching the half-century mark is a milestone. Being powerful and in control can count against us, causing us to make assumptions and jump to premature conclusions.

In our culture, it is OK to have a little meat on your bones. Caucasian women have traditionally been under more pressure to appear youthful and thin, leading to feelings of apprehension about aging, which can aggravate their symptoms during menopause. I have found that Caucasian women tend to be more worried about those first few wrinkles that appear at age forty than we are. Like they say, "Black don't crack." But some of us still have fears about what happens to us midlife because we are not happy with the courses our lives have taken.

> **"Whatever you fear, most fears have no power, it is your fear that has the power."**
> —*Oprah Winfrey*

Increase Your Knowledge About Cultural Attitudes Regarding Women and Aging

As you increase your knowledge about your options for treatment, take some time to explore what other cultures have to say about aging women.

Conduct your own anthropological study of how our culture treats older women.

ARE YOU IN A DOWNWARD SPIRAL ABOUT MENOPAUSE?

If we find ourselves bombarded with symptoms that affect our functioning, such as mood swings and loss of memory, we could fall into a downward spiral about menopause. We may find ourselves in a rut due to the overwhelming nature of some of our symptoms and the impact of any negative feelings we harbor about maturing. On the other hand, some Black women report that they expect menopause to be easy. This transition fills them with a sense of freedom. Their mothers breezed through, and they expect to do the same. They have a mindset geared toward an easy transition because that has been the family experience. What our mothers say and do is an important factor in determining our attitudes about menopause, just as they are important in determining attitudes relating to other developmental stages.

SELF-EFFICACY

Theories and principles from so-called self-help and pop psychology provide tools to help us reinvent ourselves. Learning more about self-efficacy and how to increase it will help us change our attitudes, assumptions, and beliefs about what we are capable of achieving in the Second Half of Life.

> **"There is no more creative force in the world than the menopausal woman with zest."**
>
> —*Margaret Mead*

Self-efficacy is defined as our attitude about our ability to make things happen in our lives, to make changes, and to achieve our goals. Dr. Albert Bandura of Stanford University began studying self-efficacy more than twenty years ago. He states, "The achievement of insight or self awareness is essential for producing enduring behavioral changes." His research indicates that self-efficacy can be improved through several techniques, including mentoring, affirmation, positive reinforcement, and visualization. Increasing self-efficacy helps you change your attitudes about menopause.

Self-efficacy helps us cope with change

When we feel efficacious, we are strong, productive, and confident about being in control of our lives. Highly efficacious people are always focusing on targets, moving forward, and overcoming challenges. Low self-efficacy is experienced when you feel that your life is controlled by outside forces. Inefficacious people are basically in a rut and don't see any way to make things better for themselves. They see themselves as powerless.

Dr. Bandura's basic premise is that self-efficacy is a learned behavior, and he believes that self-help programs are started by people who have enough self-efficacy to believe that they can make changes in their lives.

Let's look at several of these previously mentioned methods for changing your attitude about menopause and increasing your level of self-efficacy.

Mentoring

One strategy for increasing self-efficacy is to have someone who truly respects you persuade you to believe that you can make wonderful changes. We can all probably remember when someone close to us had more faith in our ability to succeed than we did. This is one of the reasons that mentoring works. Mentors usually have very high expectations of the people they are mentoring.

I had several older "sister" role models who inspired me to believe that menopause is a new beginning. My mother is a very active and still beautiful woman who has never let aging become a negative factor in her life. My aunts Marie and Olivia believe they are only getting better and life has more in store for them. Aunt Marie says, "I have never worried about getting older. I love my life and look forward to every day. I feel blessed to be here and I haven't lost a thing." My dear friend Floretta is a vibrant and beautiful woman who has a zest for life and is a joy to be around. Being eighty years old has given her more wisdom to share with others. These wonderful women have mentored me and helped me increase my level of self-efficacy.

Affirmations and self-efficacy

Affirming that you are powerful increases self-efficacy. Affirmations are powerful, one-sentence goal-oriented statements that you use to bring about different results in your life. They work because they impact our subconscious mind. Whatever we say, the subconscious mind believes. This process can work to our success or to our failure because when we think negative thoughts or put ourselves down, we are affirming negative thoughts and goals. Affirmations help us program our subconscious mind to focus on positive thoughts tied to our goals. We begin to change by intent and move in the direction we choose. We become more self-directed. Since we have about fifty thousand thoughts a day, it makes sense to work on directing those thoughts as much as we can toward the things we want.

Rules for writing affirmations

- ◆ Affirmations should be positive
- ◆ They must be personal. You can only affirm for yourself
- ◆ Write them in the present tense
- ◆ Make them clear and specific
- ◆ Use words that express movement, enthusiasm, and excitement
- ◆ Avoid words and phrases such as "should," "could," "will," "can," and "I intend to." These words cause us to procrastinate

Answer the following questions and write your affirmations based on the way you want things to be.

+ What am I thinking about perimenopause/menopause?
+ How do I want to think about perimenopause/menopause?
+ What thoughts, images, and pictures would help me see this transition differently, and how can I affirm a new picture or attitude?

AFFIRMATIONS

* I am a healthy, strong, and powerful African-American woman.
* I thrive on the changes taking place in my body and I am successful in changing my mind about this transition.
* Perimenopause/menopause is a wonderful phase of life for me.
* I am enjoying each aspect of my exciting transition.

Visualization

After you affirm the way you want your transition to be, the next step is to practice visualizing your Second Half of Life. Making use of the wonderful power of your imagination is an effective method for increasing self-efficacy and personal power. Direct the pictures in your mind based on what you want and the way you want things to be. It is a natural process because it is our nature to move toward our goals. We are attracted to the pictures and images we hold in our minds.

MENOPAUSE CALL TO ACTION

+ Take responsibility for your menopause.
+ Develop a new passion for your life and the contributions you can make to the world.

- Develop a greater sense of self-reliance.
- Create the solutions to your challenges with a sense of open-mindedness.
- Be prepared to navigate change.
- Be bold.
- Don't deny menopause—embrace it!
- Use the positive strategies passed down through generations of strong African-American women.
- Use the courage of your convictions to blast off to a new future.
- Live the life of your dreams. Don't be afraid to go all out for what you want.

CHAPTER 2

Explore Your Options: What's Going On?

I am an African-American woman who felt empowered to educate myself and explore all of my options during menopause. For years, I believed the medical profession didn't understand or care about the health issues of women. In my experience, doctors have often been unable to relate to me in a way that's culturally relevant. In other words, they didn't appear to have an understanding of what it's like to be an African-American woman.

It's also a fact that our risk factors in midlife are different. We are twice as likely as white women to develop hypertension, coronary heart disease, and diabetes after age forty. Because I see myself as powerful and have an "I can fix it" attitude, I tried to fix my menopausal journey. I had to learn that there are no quick fixes. I realized if I didn't take time to gather the appropriate information, I wouldn't know where to begin. I had to engage myself in the learning process, including learning about my health risks, understanding the conditions surrounding midlife transition, and figuring out what I needed to do to take care of myself.

I overcame my state of denial in order to face the reality of menopause and maintain an open mind about the physical, mental, and spiritual healing process that takes place during midlife. Things came to a head as I began to face my own mortality, and issues regarding my willingness to make a commitment to being well could no longer be ignored. I reached a point where I couldn't keep postponing a reckoning with lifestyle choices that had been detrimental to my wellness.

As I faced the dilemma concerning the pros and cons of hormone replacement, it was important to explore my options in a way that was culturally appropriate. I was not concerned about looking younger or getting rid of wrinkles. My priority was to determine how hormone replacement therapy would help me function effectively in spite of symptoms like hot flashes and insomnia. I did not view estrogen as a fountain of youth, but as a tool to help me maintain the quality of my life. Grappling with issues surrounding nutrition, exercise, and stress management also became imperative during this transition.

I am committed to helping Black women realize our age-related risk factors for developing certain debilitating diseases. There are many questions to be considered. Why are African-American women more prone to poor health at age fifty? What are Black women doing about their menopause symptoms? Why do we perceive breast cancer as our biggest risk factor when the probability of developing heart disease is much higher? These are some of the questions I sought to answer as I learned how to navigate this passage.

As I reflected on these questions and thought about our history, I became even more dedicated to being healthy and well during menopause. As my good friend Natilyne says, "We've been making it by on youth, but now we are going to have to start taking care of ourselves." In order to figure out what was best, I needed to check out all my alternatives for treating my symptoms. Midlife transition forced me to face the inevitable: my poor health decisions were catching up with me.

Minimizing our risk of developing heart disease, diabetes, and osteoporosis will have a significant impact on how well we age because these conditions are all modifiable by lifestyle choices. We have coping strategies and habitual ways of thinking and behaving that influence this mix of factors. Like many African-American women, I don't allow anyone to tell me what to do or suggest they know what's best for me. We look out for what we think is in our own best interest even when we don't have the knowledge to do so. One such thought pattern we adhere to is "I can take care of this by myself." However, this typical response just didn't cut it during menopause. I couldn't just zip through it. I had to invent a path for moving through the changes in a thoughtful, conscious manner that made sense for a healthier lifestyle. That is our common task.

Another barrier was my lack of trust in the medical establishment. Our cultural background and history has led many of us to become very skeptical of medical research. The aftereffects of the Tuskegee Project are still causing me and many other African-Americans to distrust the positive results of what medical science has to offer. In this study, which took place several decades ago, African-American men who tested positive for syphilis were denied treatment. They were used as guinea pigs to track the progress of this debilitating disease, which could have been easily cured with penicillin. When the true facts were released and people learned about the horrible deed that was done, Black people became even more distrustful of white doctors.

I know I was too quick to prejudge my primary caregivers in a negative fashion when I should have known better, as I've been subjected to stereotypes my entire life. Although some level of distrust was justified based on my own personal experiences in the past, I am getting over it. I am prepared to give each new medical relationship the opportunity to be positive. My strategy today is to ask a lot of questions about any treatment and to do my homework. I listen to what I am told, and then I make a decision to follow the plan or not.

Dr. Levy's Perspective

As we mature and enter the perimenopausal and menopausal times in our lives, women are at an ever-increasing risk of developing cardiovascular disease, breast cancer, diabetes, and osteoporosis. African-American women have hereditary advantages in some arenas and significant disadvantages in others. The incidence of obesity and high blood pressure is significantly higher in African-American women than in the general population. These conditions can lead to a serious risk of coronary artery disease and heart attack. Unfortunately, since African-American women make up only a small number of patients in most medical studies, it is often difficult to assess the magnitude and contribution of specific risk factors to overall health.

We do know that African-American women have a lower risk of breast cancer compared to Caucasian women; however, the risk of dying from that cancer is higher for African-American women! We don't know whether that is due to decreased access to care, decreased tendency to get chemotherapy and radiation therapy, or whether the type of cancer that African-American women get is substantially more aggressive. We need answers to these questions before we can come up with strategies to decrease the death rate for African-American women from breast cancer.

Similarly, we know that the risk of obesity and diabetes is quite high in African-American women. Treatments developed and tested on Caucasian women, however, often don't work well for women of color. Our genetic makeup is quite unique and clearly influences the cause and therefore the proper treatment of these conditions. African-American women have a lower risk, in general, for osteoporosis since, genetically, their bones are denser. However, without exercise, appropriate vitamins, and calcium, African-American women do develop osteoporosis. Both African-American women and health care providers caring for them must be aware of these problems so that optimal health during the menopausal years can be achieved.

AFRICAN-AMERICAN WOMEN AND WEIGHT

Black women are much more likely to be overweight at midlife. According to Weaver, Gaines, and Ebron in *Slim Down Sister,* there are 17.8 million Black women in the United States, and approximately nine million are risking their lives each day by being overweight. They state that 52 percent of Black women are obese. Obesity is defined as being more than 20 percent overweight. I don't know about you, but for me, worrying about being overweight became a big issue for me when I turned forty. For the first time in my life, I was significantly overweight by as much as twenty-five pounds. I know we understand that we have issues with weight, but many of us are unwilling to change our habits and develop long-term solutions to the problem. Also, we may suffer from poor "body esteem," according to bell hooks in *Sisters of the Yam*. She says we need to love ourselves more so that we will take care of our bodies, but she also says we shouldn't hate ourselves because we are overweight. Self-hatred leads to another vicious cycle where we get into the rut of thinking we are worthless.

Research states that low-income, urban, African-American women have some of the highest rates of obesity in the United States. More than 10 percent of African-American women between the ages of forty and fifty-nine have a very high level of obesity. The factors leading to weight gain include cultural norms, traditions, and the way we view ourselves. Many of us have an unrealistic view of what we should weigh and have not incorporated good eating habits or regular exercise into our daily lives. We don't focus on preventing weight gain, and many of us are unaware of the serious complications tied to obesity. When the aging process begins to take a toll and our metabolism slows down, we find ourselves losing control. The typical twenty pounds that we are always trying to lose becomes fifty pounds or more. We also need to increase our knowledge about aging. Completing an assessment on these indicators will help us get a reading on how fast we are aging:

- Strength and endurance
- Basal metabolic rate
- Body-fat percentage
- Aerobic capacity
- Blood pressure
- Blood-sugar sensitivity
- Cholesterol levels
- Bone density
- Body-temperature regulation

MAKING THE TRANSITION

I had trouble recognizing when I was in perimenopause, that time when my ovaries began to decrease estrogen production. I experienced irregular menstrual cycles and erratic mood swings.

Perimenopause can be quite confusing. It is the beginning of the continuum of midlife transition. Our symptoms can be varied but subtle, or upsetting and intense. The range of symptoms is so wide that it is hard to believe they are related. Many of my friends didn't have a clue about what was going on with their bodies and couldn't advise me. Those who suspected they were starting menopause and had some inkling about what was going on would say quite emphatically, "I don't even want to hear about anything with the word menopause attached to it." I hear them and I feel them because I know what it feels like to want to postpone the inevitable. We may not want to go there, but Mother Nature is telling us it is time. Menopause hasn't caused me to age, but not taking care of my health will age me.

Perimenopause begins when your body decreases estrogen production. The symptoms include irregular periods, mood swings, lack of elasticity in tissues such as the vagina, fatigue, changes in sexual desire, dry skin, underactive thyroid, sleep disturbances, heavy bleeding, memory lapses, reduced muscle tone, eye dryness, and reduced vitality. African-American women report that irregular periods and heavy bleeding are among the early symptoms. They report, "I went from having regular periods to having a cycle every twenty-one days to forty-two days. I never knew when it was going to come."

Sometimes it's really hard to believe that you are starting the transition. Kim, for example, had no idea that perimenopause can start seven to ten years before menopause. A thirty-eight-year-old African-American woman, Kim had been experiencing slightly irregular periods, heavy flow, pain with her period, mood swings, urinary-tract infections, and very dry skin. She did not believe that this was the beginning of menopause, even though her sister suggested it. She also discussed her symptoms with her mother, who told her she experienced similar symptoms when she was forty-two. Her mother took Premarin, an estrogen pill, for five years in her late forties and early fifties. Kim's periods come every twenty to forty days and she is overweight. She has a family history of high blood pressure. Her blood pressure was borderline high at 142/85. To determine the onset of menopause, a follicle stimulating hormone test was completed, and it revealed that perimenopause had begun. She started taking low-dosage, plant-based estrogen tablets, which took care of her symptoms. She started a regular exercise plan and a low-fat, low-sodium diet. She now feels wonderful and is back in control of her life.

AFRICAN-AMERICAN WOMEN AND ESTROGEN USE

It's hard to think about menopause without talking about what we know about estrogen. African-American women are less likely to use estrogen to slow down aging. Approximately 46 percent of African American women report estrogen-related symptoms such as flashes, vaginal dryness, memory problems, poor coordination, dizziness, and night sweats. African-American women are less willing to participate in research studies on estrogen use and generally have less knowledge about hormone replacement therapy (HRT). African-American women are more likely to be concerned about the risk of cancer as a possible side effect of HRT. They tend to view menopause as a normal phase and therefore don't see a need to be treated for their symptoms.

There are many myths about the use of estrogen, including:

♦ It keeps you from aging.

♦ It makes you retain water.

♦ It will keep you from getting wrinkles.

♦ It makes you fat.

♦ It causes breast cancer or uterine cancer.

♦ If we needed estrogen after age fifty, our bodies would still produce it.

Focusing on these myths will cause us to overestimate the consequences of diminishing hormones in midlife. It makes more sense to gather accurate information and address our fears.

As I prepared for menopause, I read everything I could find about the pros and cons of using estrogen. Dr. Levy answered all my questions and helped me to see that because my menopause was surgically induced, my situation was different. Those of us who have had our uteruses and/or ovaries removed have no choice about using estrogen, at least for a short period of time. It is too traumatic for the body to adjust to such an abrupt lack of estrogen with no replacement. Black women going through natural menopause have more time for their bodies to adjust to diminishing levels of estrogen.

After a while, I considered myself well-educated on menopause and found some of my strategies to be quite successful. I was very diligent about exercising and eating properly and lost twenty-seven pounds in the six months following my hysterectomy. I felt more in control and began to believe everything else would happen according to my plans.

I was in for a rude awakening! I was prepared for my hysterectomy surgery, but I was not totally prepared for menopause. All of my lifestyle changes and strategies were helpful, but I still experienced hot flashes, depression, mood swings, memory loss, insomnia, and the inability to concentrate. It took time to develop the right combination of strategies, and I had to learn to be diligent, persistent, and patient. Early in my transition, I was so resistant to taking any estrogen that I only agreed to a low-dose estrogen patch that helped diminish but did not alleviate my symptoms. Dr. Levy, concerned about my past history of having endometriosis, a condition where uterine tissues grow outside the uterus, was also in favor of a low dosage.

As it turned out, my most severe symptom was insomnia, and it caught me off guard. No one had prepared me for this. None of the resources I used led me to believe that it was possible to lose my ability to sleep because of a lack of estrogen. My first response was to go into warrior mode and treat this hurdle as a battle, but eventually I stepped back and thought more about healing.

I used self-care methods, which we Black women are prone to do. I got massages, took long baths, and listened to my favorite music to relax. It's part of our culture to do what we can to take care of things on our own. My strategies also included experimenting with herbs and over-the-counter sleep remedies. Nothing helped me sleep more than two or three hours per night.

I had control of my work schedule and adjusted my hours because I couldn't manage getting to work before 11 A.M. and usually worked until 5 or 6 P.M. My ability to concentrate was impaired, and sometimes I couldn't force myself to complete projects. This was not like me, as I am usually a master at juggling numerous projects. I turned down an exciting training opportunity during this time when someone called me at the last moment and wanted me to start a new contract with very little time to prepare. For the first time, I just couldn't rise to the challenge. I was afraid and filled with self-doubt. It was a crisis of confidence. At other times, I felt euphoric and extremely confident. I experienced a see-saw of emotions.

Sometimes, I would get sleepy in the afternoon and come home hoping to take a nap, but I was never able to do so during those months. Ironically, in my family I was known as the "Queen of Sleep." I have always been able to fall asleep at the drop of a hat for ten minutes or several hours.

After increasing my estrogen to a higher dosage, I recaptured my ability to sleep for a full eight hours. I learned another important lesson: natural remedies are helpful, but when you have a serious hormonal imbalance, you need to see natural remedies as only one component of your treatment plan.

In the midst of all of this, I started a very stressful project. I was commuting from Seattle to Detroit two to three times per month to fulfill a large contract. As executive director of a large employment and training project, I had to spend eight to ten days per month supervising a staff of ten and overseeing the delivery of motivational training and job-development services to unemployed people. This was the largest contract in the history of our company, L.L. Brown International, Inc., and also the most stressful for many reasons. Finally, I decided, and my husband Lester and my financial advisor both agreed with me, that it was time to pack it in.

Before my surgery, Les and I had several conversations about my health. I told him that my periods were out of control and I that was going to have to do something drastic soon. He kept saying, "If you need surgery, just go ahead and get it." I knew he was right when we traveled to London and

Scotland that year to help our newest distributor expand her contracts. My period came two weeks early, and I was in the bathroom every thirty to forty-five minutes for seven days. When you are in a foreign country dealing with a problem like this, it really is a nightmare. I was embarrassed about constantly needing to go to the restroom and was often in a panic trying to find one in unfamiliar buildings.

I explained to my husband that having a hysterectomy was a major undertaking because it would throw me into menopause immediately, but I knew he didn't really understand. I knew menopause was going to take me on a path requiring major adjustments in my life. I also knew it was going to be difficult for him because he had never seen me go through any major physical or emotional changes. He depended on me to write new workbooks and develop new markets while he was on the road delivering services and creating leads. I had been playing the role of the strong African-American woman for so long that neither of us could imagine what it would be like for me to take some down time. I remember telling my staff that I would be back to work in two weeks. I was very unrealistic and was still trying to control everything. I refused to slow down and think about how I was feeling. I didn't want to know what was going on. I believe in "possibility thinking," that adversity provides an opportunity, but the healing process cannot be rushed.

Once I began this journey, I felt so vulnerable. Les tried to understand how I felt, but often I didn't even know myself. My cultural conditioning about being a strong woman was crucial to my self-image and personal success. I believed that strong women don't complain, they just take care of business and do what needs to be done. In the beginning stages of menopause, my greatest strength became my greatest weakness because I was so determined to do it my way. Then I realized it was time for me to redefine my purpose in life and to make a total commitment to taking care of myself. I stopped being so driven and became more in tune with myself and listened to the messages that my body was giving me.

I know now that menopause should be celebrated and that it can be the best time of our lives. I am excited and thrilled about what I have been able to accomplish in the years since I began this transition. I really feel like I have it going on. I feel absolutely wonderful and now I see things with such clarity. It's easier for me to do what I need to do for myself and I have more inner peace, wisdom, and knowledge to share with you. I offer myself and my experiences as a mirror to help you, my sisters, take a closer look at your transition and your life.

Many African-American women report experiencing the beginning of hormonal changes in their late thirties and early forties, as I did. Although irregular bleeding is quite often our first symptom of perimenopause, some women have their last cycle without any warning or noticeable changes. They don't realize the significance of tracking their monthly cycles as they get closer to age fifty. I counsel a lot of women who are desperate for guidance and accurate information. They complain because their employers don't provide employee assistance in this area and they have to struggle to find resources on their own. Some are frustrated because they try talking to friends who get defensive and don't want to face their own transition. When they approach their doctors, they are sometimes told that they are too young and their symptoms must be stress-related.

A small percentage of African-American women experience menopause before the age of forty due to hereditary factors, problems with their immune systems, cancer treatment, hormonal disorders, and complications from childhood illnesses such as mumps or viral infections. I find many of us don't have a clue about when we will start or what factors influence the onset of menopause.

What's the Big Deal About Estrogen?

Whenever the word "menopause" is mentioned, the first question asked is usually related to whether or not estrogen replacement is necessary. Everyone wants to know why estrogen is such a big deal. It is because estrogen is one of the most important hormones in a woman's body. From the time of our first periods to our last, our ovaries produce estrogen. Imbalances occur when estrogen levels fluctuate and production varies. During a woman's lifespan, this type of imbalance typically occurs during puberty and menopause along with other physiological and psychological changes.

Estrogen affects more than three hundred tissues in a woman's body, including the brain, vagina, bones, blood vessels, urinary tract, gastrointestinal tract, breasts, and skin. The endocrine system, which is responsible for metabolism, growth, and reproduction, is also affected. Estrogen receptors, those sites in a woman's body where estrogen is supposed to enter like a key into a lock, have been found throughout our bodies, indicating that estrogen is meant to bind or attach itself at these locations. Menopause begins when there isn't enough estrogen produced to make our uterine lining grow.

Dr. Levy explains how many of the physical changes we experience are related to hormonal changes. "Actually," she says, "female hormones are constantly changing from birth until after menopause. Sometimes our lives have more constant or stable levels of hormones while others are more variable and the levels go up and down. Certainly, the time between ages thirty and thirty-five to fifty are as variable as adolescence, ages eight to sixteen. The changes that accompany these time periods are important because they help us understand what's happening to our bodies. The beginning phase of all these changes usually starts about age thirty-eight to forty-three, although this varies for different women. Our goal is to become more aware of these fluxes—socially, emotionally, and hormonally."

As we expand our knowledge about estrogen, we begin to understand why there is so much discussion about this hormone. Whether we decide to use synthetic estrogen, natural estrogen, or herbal remedies that mimic estrogen in our bodies, estrogen plays many roles. There has been a lot of negative and often confusing information released about hormone replacement therapy that implies doctors and drug companies have been pushing estrogen on women since the 1940s and 1950s. People who support this view point out that at one time almost all women were put on a standard regimen of Premarin .625, the most widely prescribed form of estrogen pill. Many women who still had a uterus developed problems because they were not given estrogen in combination with progesterone. Nowadays, estrogen is always prescribed in combination with progesterone for women who retain their uteruses.

In the past, there has been very little research available on women and aging, especially African-American women. Today, as a result of new information, many doctors are more than willing to work with their patients in a partnership to determine if estrogen is necessary and the best form or dosage. Many factors are taken into consideration before a decision is made. Hormone replacement is not necessary for all women. Each one of us is different, but there is a need to discuss our symptoms in great detail along with our medical history, including our reproductive medical history. We must engage in a dialogue that will help determine what we need. It is also important to talk about our emotional needs and our stressors, even if it goes against our beliefs about "not putting our business in the streets."

African-American women who are not in the habit of asking for help or who may not be working with a culturally competent primary caregiver may need to pay special attention to clearly stating their needs and documenting their symptoms and feelings. Since we tend to see each new phase of our life as a battle, we communicate our situation by talking about how we intend to overcome the challenge without clearly telling our caregiver what we are experiencing. Some caregivers don't understand the necessity of probing for a better description of our symptoms. Our method of communicating in combination with our strong sense of self makes them think we have everything under control. Keeping a menopause journal to share with our doctors will help us describe what's going on and will improve communication, thereby assisting the decision-making process.

WHAT'S GOING ON WITH US DURING MENOPAUSE?

You probably know what I'm talking about when I say many African-American women report gaining weight during and after menopause without any increase in food consumption or changes in the diet. Almost all of us report feelings of anxiety and stress because our bodies change and we don't know what to expect. Each day is like charting new territory.

For example, estrogen, or lack of it, may result in short-term memory loss and "fuzzy" thinking, which are quite common, along with a lack of concentration and focus. We find it difficult to function up to our normal levels at home and at work, but most of us summon up enough energy to maintain the status quo. However, everything seems harder. Maybe you have experienced the following: Do you find it more difficult to do five things at once and keep a mental picture of your schedule? Has it become imperative to write things down? Dr. Levy tells us doctors don't know why this happens, but that they have heard it from enough women to realize that estrogen or lack of estrogen definitely affects parts of the brain and certain aspects of our cognitive ability.

Symptoms of menopause

♦ Hot flashes
♦ Poor memory

- ◆ Headaches
- ◆ Vaginal dryness
- ◆ Decreased libido
- ◆ Backache
- ◆ Decreased self-esteem
- ◆ Insomnia
- ◆ Depression
- ◆ Inability to concentrate
- ◆ Mood swings
- ◆ Muscle or heel pain
- ◆ Increase in facial hair
- ◆ Joint pain
- ◆ Bladder problems
- ◆ Weight gain
- ◆ Fatigue
- ◆ Lack of energy
- ◆ Poor coordination
- ◆ Joint pain
- ◆ Urine leakage
- ◆ Reduced stamina
- ◆ Eye dryness

COPING WITH MENOPAUSE

What are our general health practices as African-American women in midlife and how can this information be used to help us and help our caregivers understand how to treat us? Researchers believe answering this question will provide us with crucial information.

We tend to go to family members or our support network when we are confronted with challenges, including menopause. We believe in self-care as the first defense. Self-care is good, but we need to recognize when professional help is required. Our level of knowledge about our conditions and risk factors is limited and often we are very sick by the time we seek the help of a doctor. Often we don't have access to accurate information or we don't trust the sources. Levels of education and income are factors that influence whether or not we, African-American women, have access to accurate medical information about menopause.

Many African-American women tell me their hot flashes last from a few seconds to several minutes. They report feeling extremely warm and sweaty all over, but mostly in the upper body or on their thighs. Some flash throughout the day and others experience only night sweats. Sometimes our symptoms come all at once and it is hard to ignore them, even though it may take us a while before we do anything about them.

Did you know...

Did you know 66 percent of all women experience mild to extreme hot flashes during menopause?

Did you know most hot flashes last for one minute or less?

Did you know chemotherapy, radiation treatment, and pelvic surgery can contribute to early menopause?

Did you know there will be fifty million women in menopause by 2005 and approximately seven million will be African-American?

TESTOSTERONE

Testosterone is another sex hormone we need to know about as it may decrease during menopause. A deficiency of this hormone, which is an androgen, can negatively impact our menopausal journey. It is associated with a loss of drive, energy, sexual desire, and thinning pubic hair. If you have a deficiency, testosterone can be supplemented in small doses of cream or gel. Some Black women say they are afraid of testosterone because they have been told it makes you act like a man. I reassure them that this is not true, as our bodies have always produced a certain amount of it. Talk with your health care provider to pinpoint if you are experiencing diminished vitality and sexual response. Don't hesitate to check it out!

CHAPTER 3

Get Educated: Know What You Need to Know

We've been defining menopause and how it feels; now let's get educated. A review of information about hormone replacement therapy, osteoporosis, coronary heart disease, breast cancer, and diabetes helps us explore the long-term health consequences of menopause. Each condition can lead to serious problems and each has the potential to negatively impact our standard of living. Increasing our knowledge about these conditions, and exploring prevention strategies, will help us maintain good health.

OSTEOPOROSIS

Osteoporosis is a serious health risk for women once they reach menopause because loss of estrogen leads to weaker bones. Most women begin losing bone mass around age thirty-five. This bone loss leads to osteoporosis when bones become very brittle and begin to break easily. Fractures in the back (vertebrae) cause women to have humps in their backs and lose height. Hip fractures are most devastating because the ability to move around and be independent is severely limited.

Until recently, we have been told our risks for osteoporosis were practically nonexistent. But new studies show that there are more than three hundred thousand cases of Black women with osteoporosis documented in the last five years. That number of cases could increase once African-American women and their doctors become more aware of the level of risk and African-American women are more routinely tested, according to Cathy R. Kessenids at the Tampa University School of Nursing.

Unfortunately, osteoporosis is a silent disease and there are no symptoms until a bone is broken. It does not cause pain. Osteoporosis cannot be cured, but it can be prevented. The best test for assessing osteoporosis is the bone mineral densitometry test. A DEXA scanner, a special type of X ray machine, is used to determine the level of bone mass by measuring at your hip, vertebrae, and lower arm.

Some African-American women may be at higher risk for developing osteoporosis because they are underweight and have a small frame. Take Gwen, for example, a fifty-year-old African-American woman who is experiencing flashes and irritability. She had her last period nine months ago. She works out religiously but does not eat properly and is fifteen pounds underweight. She had a myomectomy, a procedure to remove non-cancerous tumors from the uterus, at age thirty-eight, and has had no recurring fibroids (tumors on her uterus). She has a family history of hysterectomy, usually by age forty-five. Her periods were regular, but then stopped after missing a period two to three times per year for about two years. She eats lots of soy and took several over-the-counter menopausal herbal remedies. She received some relief for a while, but her hot flashes were starting to interfere with her sex and work lives. Also, because of her size and bone structure, she was told she might be at risk for osteoporosis. She was given a low-dosage estrogen patch with progestin, a form of progesterone to protect the lining of her uterus. She was encouraged to eat balanced meals with lots of fruit and vegetables and to take 1200 mg of calcium with magnesium.

MENOPAUSE STRATEGIES

There are several things that we can do to prevent bone loss, such as taking adequate calcium and vitamin D and eating leafy green vegetables such as collard greens, mustard greens, and turnip greens, all of which provide calcium. Low-fat dairy products, beans, and fish are also excellent sources of calcium. Historically, African-American women have always eaten greens as a staple of the traditional "soul food" diet. Our grandparents had a lifestyle that helped them get adequate calcium. They grew their own vegetables, raised grain-fed chickens and cattle, and made their own cheese, butter, and ice cream. Everything they cooked was fresh and free of preservatives. Some of us have gotten away from eating these homegrown, natural foods.

The progress of osteoporosis can be stopped, and bone loss can be restored with hormone treatment. There are other treatment options available for women who can't take estrogen such as alendronate (Fosamax) and calcitonin (Miacalcin).

Osteoporosis Risk Factors

- ◆ Family history
- ◆ Low-calcium diet
- ◆ Fair hair
- ◆ Cigarette smoking
- ◆ Alcohol abuse
- ◆ Early menopause
- ◆ Use of medications, such as corticosteriods
- ◆ Slender build
- ◆ Prolonged absence of period
- ◆ Lactose intolerance
- ◆ Vitamin D deficiency

♦ Lack of exercise
♦ Thyroid disease

What is your level of risk?

Rate yourself. If you have more than five of the factors listed above, you may be at risk for developing osteoporosis. We recommend that you take calcium supplements even though there is no research on how African-American women respond to calcium supplementation.

Did You Know...

Did you know as many as 75 percent of African-Americans are lactose intolerant, which makes it difficult for them to get sufficient calcium through their diet?

Did you know once estrogen production decreases, bone loss occurs at a rate as high as 7 percent per year?

Did you know 20 percent of women who break a hip die within one year?

BREAST CANCER

Fear of breast cancer is one of the main reasons many African-American women resist taking estrogen during menopause. However, taking estrogen does not automatically lead to an increased risk of breast cancer. Women who have a family history of breast cancer should be cautious in making decisions about estrogen replacement therapy or hormone replacement therapy.

In 1964, there was a one in twenty chance of developing breast cancer in this country. At age forty today, there is a one in twenty-three chance of developing breast cancer. The chances increase with age. The good news is that breast cancer rates dropped 5 percent between 1989 and 1993. African-American women have a higher mortality rate for breast cancer due to several factors, including late detection. Our cancers tend to be detected at a more advanced stage. We may underestimate our risk of breast cancer, believing that previous medical history is the major risk factor when in fact 80 percent of women who have breast cancer have no previous family medical history.

Every woman should make it a priority to know her risk of developing breast cancer.

Breast cancer risk factors
Being over the age of fifty is the major factor for breast cancer. Others include:
+ Family history of breast cancer
+ Having your first child after age thirty
+ No children
+ High-fat diet
+ Obesity, especially in your upper body
+ Starting menstruation before the age of eleven
+ Smoking
+ Lumps or pain in the previous six months
+ Obesity

Breast cancer symptoms
+ A change in the size of the breast
+ A lump in the breast
+ Breast discharge
+ A change in coloring of the skin or nipple
+ A change in the skin of the breast

It is also encouraging to note that more than 90 percent of the women who develop breast cancer survive. However, this statistic does not hold true for African-American women, as we are less likely to conduct our monthly exams and get mammograms.

There are Black women who have survived breast cancer, such as Joyce, fifty-two, an African-American woman who has been cancer-free for six years. A masectomy was not required, but she had chemotherapy. She is suffering from hot flashes, mood swings, and poor memory, and she has tried several herbal remedies, including black cohosh, evening primrose oil, and raspberry leaf with minimal relief. She is forty pounds overweight and has not had a period since she began chemotherapy. Her first marriage ended in divorce and her second husband died after seven years of marriage. She is very happy in her third marriage. Joyce was asked to work out four times per week for one hour and has started a weight-loss program focusing on losing two pounds per week. She is using Vivelle, an estrogen skin patch for the hot flashes and using an estrogen ring for vaginal dryness. Joyce is pleased with the results she's getting and is well on her way to celebrating the Second Half of Life.

Breast Cancer Prevention

The following tips can help to prevent breast cancer or detect it early:

- ♦ Give yourself a monthly breast exam.
- ♦ Eat a high-fiber diet with a lot of vegetables like greens, cabbage, spinach, carrots, and yams. Eat like our grandmothers!
- ♦ Add soy products to your diet.
- ♦ Make it a habit to exercise three to four times per week for at least thirty minutes.
- ♦ Have a mammogram once a year.
- ♦ Learn some type of formal method of relaxation like meditation, autohypnosis, or progressive muscle relaxation.
- ♦ Manage stress effectively.

CORONARY HEART DISEASE

Coronary heart disease causes 50 percent of all deaths of women over the age of fifty and is the leading cause of death for Black people. It becomes an issue for all women because we are more susceptible to this disease once our estrogen levels decrease. The current belief is that estrogen may provide some protection against heart disease, but many African-American women don't understand how or why estrogen might be of benefit to them.

Coronary heart disease (CHD) can start developing even in children as fat-like substances build up on the walls of our blood vessels and cause them to harden and narrow. This decreases the flow of blood to the heart, which can lead to chest pain. Whenever blood flow is restricted, a heart attack can occur. The research is conflicting, but some studies show that women who take estrogen during menopause show a significant reduction in the likelihood of developing CHD.

Coronary heart disease risk factors

+ Being over the age of fifty-five
+ Having a family history of heart disease
+ Being overweight
+ A lack of exercise
+ Diabetes
+ High blood pressure
+ High cholesterol
+ Being a smoker

A family medical history of heart disease is a reality for Sheila, a forty-five-year-old African-American woman who had been experiencing hot flashes and night sweats almost every night for six months. She also had trouble sleeping even when she wasn't flashing. Her periods were regular but she had heavy flow with clots. She has a family history of fibroids and hysterectomy. Her mother had surgery at age thirty-nine but retained her ovaries. She also has a family history of breast cancer and heart disease, although her blood pressure is normal at 118/76. Sheila smokes fifteen cigarettes daily and did not realize smoking is a factor for early menopause. She has wanted to quit for years but was afraid of gaining weight. She took birth-control pills for ten years but is now using a sponge and condom. She was given a combination low-dosage estrogen tablet with progestin (to protect against endometrial cancer) and was advised to stop smoking immediately. She began exercising three times each week and switched to a low-fat diet to minimize weight gain. Her symptoms have been alleviated and she only gained five pounds when she quit smoking.

Coronary heart disease can be detected in the following ways:

♦ **Stress test (on the treadmill):** measures what happens when more effort is needed from the heart muscle
♦ **Electrocardiogram (EKG):** detects abnormal heartbeats, blood flow, and heart-muscle damage
♦ **Coronary Angiography:** a catheter through the arteries in the arm or leg that squirts dye and detects blockages
♦ **Echocardiography:** sound waves used to detect how much blood the arteries pump out

Coronary heart disease prevention

♦ Quit smoking. Smoking speeds up the hardening of your arteries.
♦ Lose weight. Obesity is a risk factor for heart disease.
♦ Lower your blood pressure by reducing fat and sodium in your diet and increasing fiber. Frequent exercise and stress control also help to lower blood pressure. High blood pressure (over 140/90) makes your heart work harder.

♦ Lower your cholesterol. High cholesterol causes plaque to build up inside the walls of your blood vessels and increases the risk of heart disease. Additional nutritional and holistic strategies for maintaining a healthy heart will be discussed in more detail in chapter 6.

AFRICAN-AMERICAN WOMEN AND HEART DISEASE

Black women who smoke double their risk of heart disease because smoking causes heart disease by damaging the blood vessels. More than 22 percent of African-American women smoke, and many don't realize the impact of smoking on developing heart disease. Black women also have a higher rate of death from heart attack and stroke than any other group of women. Almost 80 percent of African-American women over the age of sixty have high blood pressure, which is a leading indicator for heart disease. More than 50 percent of Black women are overweight, and obesity is also a major risk factor for heart disease. Obesity accounts for 33 percent of the heart attacks experienced by African-American women.

> **"We are the only category of Americans for whom heart health statistics have worsened over the last ten years."**
> —*Dr. Beverly Yates*

DIABETES

African-American women have a high risk for developing diabetes after the age of fifty. Having this disease means your body does not use glucose effectively because the pancreas fails to produce the amount of insulin needed to turn sugar into energy. Excess sugar remains in the bloodstream and causes damage to the heart, nerves, kidneys, and eyes. One of the first signs of diabetes is impaired glucose tolerance.

There are two types of diabetes. Type I means your body doesn't make insulin. Only 5 percent of African-American women have Type I diabetes. Type II means your body can't use the insulin in your system. Of special interest, diabetes is often triggered by obesity, and more than 60 percent of African-American women are overweight. African-American women with diabetes are twice as likely to develop heart disease. Approximately 25 percent of African-American women over the age of fifty-five have Type II diabetes. It is estimated that close to one million African-American women have diabetes and do not know it.

Diabetes prevention

♦ **Nutrition:** decrease fats, sugar, and carbohydrates.
♦ **Exercise:** frequent exercise helps to move sugar out of the blood.
♦ **Blood sugar level:** know your blood sugar levels. Have them measured during your annual exam, especially if you have family history of diabetes or if you are overweight.

Life Lesson

Dealing with menopause forced me to learn new habits, take charge of my health, and see my life from a different perspective. One day, I woke up and realized that I felt better than I have ever felt in my life. Managing menopause successfully is a new paradigm. Every time I thought it was time to go on with business as usual, I realized I needed to change and take care of myself on several different levels. Every time I solved one puzzle, another one surfaced. While I worked on my physical symptoms, I started doing a mental house cleaning as well. Everything is related. I faced my health issues as well as my vulnerability. That is not easy for Black women to do at any stage of life. At first I thought my body was betraying me, but it was just letting me know I needed to listen to its messages!

AFFIRMATIONS
- I value myself enough to get educated about menopause and I move through the transition with ease.
- I am resilient and bounce back from temporary setbacks during the Second Half of Life.
- My increased knowledge empowers me to make the best decisions.

Ask Dr. Levy

Q: How can you tell if you're starting menopause?

A: You can't. Remember that it is a transition. It isn't a point in time and it isn't a boundary. As we mature, the number of eggs in our ovaries diminish. Once we hit our forties, they diminish much more rapidly, so the hormonal ebbs and flows become more erratic. The ovaries continue to make lots of estrogen, but if we haven't ovulated during a particular cycle we don't make progesterone. The beginning phases of the transition to menopause are phases in which the balances between estrogen and progesterone get out of kilter, and when that balance is out of kilter our cycles may be somewhat irregular, although they may not. We may have more symptoms like breast tenderness, water retention, and irritability. A slew of new symptoms can also appear. It's really important for people to know when they do. Simply stated, this is a time of fluctuation, of ups and downs. A roller coaster is a pretty good analogy. There are great times and not-so-great times when it comes to hormones. Smoothing out the hormonal ride with a good diet, exercise, and other healthy habits can make a big difference in how you feel.

Q: What tests would you recommend for predicting menopause?

A: I recommend the follicle stimulating hormone test (FSH). This hormone tells the ovary to make eggs. In the early stages of menopause, the level of this hormone will be elevated because ovulation has slowed down or stopped.

Q: What are the signs of the beginning of the transition from premenopause to menopause?

A: The beginning stages of menopause occur when estrogen production decreases. It usually begins around age thirty-five.

Q: Tell us more about the different types of estrogen.

A: There are three primary estrogens: estradiol, estrone, and estriol. The natural estrogen as made by the ovaries is estradiol. Estradiol is a chemical formulation in the body that is then converted by different systems in the body to estrone. Fat tissues, for example, convert estradiol to estrone. Women who are overweight have higher levels of estrone. At menopause, we make more conversion to estrone from estradiol than we do in the premenopausal time frame. Estriol is an estrogen made only by the placenta during pregnancy and is only natural during pregnancy. For the most part, it is a very small proportion of the amount of estrogen we have for the rest of our lives. The theory many proponents of estriol promote is that women who have had many pregnancies or become pregnant at a young age have a lower risk of breast cancer because estriol is a safer estrogen. It's a less potent estrogen. If you take a molecule of estriol and attach it to an estrogen receptor, it possesses about a tenth of the effect a molecule of estradiol would have. So if you take enough estriol to resolve symptoms, then you're basically getting the same amount of response that you would with estradiol because the body is going to convert it however it needs to convert it. And the theory that women on the estrogen replacement therapy formulations like Triest, which are estriol dominant, do not develop breast cancer or uterine cancer is inaccurate. They do. If they are getting enough estrogen, any one of the three types, to stop symptoms, they're getting enough in theory to promote estrogen-sensitive breast cancers.

In my practice, several women on those formulations have developed breast cancer and uterine cancer. So, I think the bottom line is you cannot substitute these three different estrogens— estradiol, estrone, and estriol— for each other. They are not dose equivalent, but if you get enough of any of them to solve menopause symptoms, then you're getting enough to cause all the negative side effects.

Q: What are the pros and cons of ERT and HRT?
A: Hormone replacement therapy means estrogen and progesterone for women who have a uterus. Estrogen replacement therapy means estrogen alone for women who do not have a uterus. The most important point is, if a woman is having symptoms, we need to treat them. The reason I treat women is to help them feel better. In terms of prevention of osteoporosis and coronary heart disease, we don't know whether estrogen is preventive or not. We know that maintaining adequate estrogen will prevent osteoporosis, but that might be at the expense of some increase in breast cancer risk, while not an increase in breast cancer death due to hormone replacement therapy. I do not recommend women take hormone replacement therapy when they are sleeping well, their vaginas are moist, and they are not having any hot flashes or night sweats. I don't think it makes sense to use ERT and HRT as a preventive for heart disease. There are other medications and lifestyle changes that we can do that should do very well for people.

Q: What is the role of family history in menopause?

A: Taking a look at family history is the best measure of when you will start menopause. Earlier and late menopause tends to run in families. Even though the average age is fifty-one and one half to fifty-two, women can start at thirty-two. The onset varies a great deal, and the best way to predict what can happen to you is to learn about the experience of your older sisters, cousins, mother, and aunts. Family history helps to determine the age at which we run out of eggs. Genetically, people age at different rates. The only things we can so to influence the timing of menopause is to do to harmful things to the ovaries, like smoking and using drugs.

Q: What role does stress play in menopause?

A: Stress increases the symptoms of any condition and contributes to a low tolerance for body changes, a low pain threshold, and a lack of ovulation imbalance in hormones.

Q: Why do some women pass through menopause without hot flashes?

A: We don't really know, but healthy lifestyles, spirituality, exercise, and a balanced diet and life make people significantly more tolerant of physical symptoms.

Q: How does being overweight affect menopause?

A: Not directly, but fat tissue converts hormones made in the adrenal gland into estrogen, so theoretically overweight women should have decreased symptoms. Overweight women have a lower risk of osteoporosis. However, women who are obese often have significant underlying psychological issues that render them vulnerable to experiencing distress with hormone changes, such as depression, irritability, and sleep disturbances.

Q: If a women suspects she is menopausal, what should she track in her menopause journal?

A: Sleep patterns, medicines, pain, over-the-counter herbs, vitamins and minerals, moods, sex drive, hot flashes, bladder symptoms, weight, and diet.

Q: Many women report problems with memory, but no one has given us good information about why we develop so many problems with our memory. What's the story?

A: Researchers have not been able to document how lack of estrogen interferes with short-term memory. We know that there are a lot of estrogen receptors in the part of the brain that handles memory. We experience cognitive losses as we get older, and distinguishing those cognitive losses from the losses related to estrogen is difficult to do. We have overloaded ourselves and our memory by looking after our husbands, our children, our jobs, the sisterhood, and the church.

Q: How does estrogen replacement therapy affect sexual arousal?

A: Mind/body connection! We are not disconnected at the neck. Estrogen does increase vaginal moisture and elasticity. It increases sensation in the genitals, and also improves mood and sleep.

Plusses and negatives of hormone replacement/estrogen replacement therapy
Plusses
- ♦ Possibly plays a role in brain functioning and memory
- ♦ May provide heart disease protection
- ♦ Prevents osteoporosis
- ♦ Eliminates hot flashes and other symptoms of menopause
- ♦ Helps prevent vaginal dryness
- ♦ Helps with general functioning

- ◆ Improves sleep quality
- ◆ Helps skin retain water
- ◆ Helps urinary incontinence

Negatives

- ◆ Unopposed estrogen without progesterone promotes cancer of the lining of the uterus
- ◆ Contributes to risk of blood clots
- ◆ May increase risk of liver and gall bladder disease
- ◆ Migraine headaches may intensify
- ◆ Can bring your period back
- ◆ Some evidence for slight increase in breast cancer risk for thin women at otherwise low risk.

DELIVERY SYSTEMS

Hormone replacement therapy/estrogen replacement therapy

The estrogen we get from pills is absorbed through the bloodstream and then sent to the liver before it can be used by the body to treat menopause symptoms such as sleep disturbances and hot flashes. Estrogen taken this way circulates throughout the body and affects a lot of different tissues.

Estrogen skin patches release a constant dosage of estrogen into the bloodstream. Patches all have the same type of estrogen, but deliver the estrogen differently through the skin. Skin patches are used to treat a broad range of menopause symptoms.

Estrogen creams are inserted directly into the vagina. The estrogen is absorbed through the vaginal lining into the bloodstream to provide relief from vaginal discomfort and dryness.

The following chart lists the brand names of hormonal formulations used to treat a variety of menopause symptoms. This chart is for informational purposes only. You should consult with your doctor before making a decision.

Pills	Bi-est, Estrace, Estradiol, Estratab, Estriol, Tri-est, Premarin, Ogen, Menest, Ortho-est, Cenestin
Vaginal creams	Premarin, Estrace, Estradiol, Estrone, Ogen, Estriol
Patches	Vivelle, FemPatch, Estradiol, Estraderm, Esclim, Climara, Alora
Vaginal ring	Estring
Vaginal pill	Vagifem
Progesterone cream/gels	Crinone, Progesterone-compound pharm, Progest, Femgest
Combination estrogen/ progestin pills	Prempro, Premphase, Activella, FemHRT, Prefest
Progesterone pills	Provera, Norlutate, Amen, Aygestin, Cycrin, Curretab, Medroxyprogesterone Acetate, Prometrium, Progesterone Compounding Pharmacy
Combination patch	CombiPatch
Combination estrogen/ testosterone pill	Estratest, Estratest HS

MENOPAUSE CALL TO ACTION

♦ Educate yourself about perimenopause and menopause.
♦ Use all your resources and skills to manage menopause in an appropriate manner.
♦ Don't be afraid to ask for help.
♦ Allow your intuition about your body to tell you when you need to slow down.
♦ Be willing to change your lifestyle when it relates to taking care of your health.

CHARTING YOUR MENOPAUSE PROFILE

Family Medical History
Is there a history of the following conditions?

General Health

High blood pressure	Yes_____	No_____
Heart disease-CHD	Yes_____	No_____
Strokes-CVD	Yes_____	No_____
Diabetes	Yes_____	No_____
Breast cancer	Yes_____	No_____
Thyroid Disease	Yes_____	No_____
Liver Disease	Yes_____	No_____

Reproductive Health

Painful periods	Yes_____	No_____
Irregular periods	Yes_____	No_____
Fibroids	Yes_____	No_____
Endometriosis	Yes_____	No_____
Hormonal imbalance	Yes_____	No_____
Hysterectomy	Yes_____	No_____
Myomectomy	Yes_____	No_____

Documenting information about your general health and reproductive health will help your doctor make a determination about the best treatment plan for you. As we have discussed, there are general health risks that increase during midlife, and previous family history is important in predicting the onset of menopause. Your specific risk factors need to be taken into account as your doctor works with you to explore the best options for treatment.

Menopausal Family History

+ What are your primary symptoms?
+ When did they start?
+ What is the intensity and duration of your symptoms?
+ How has your life been affected by perimenopause and menopause?
+ What are the primary menopausal symptoms of your relatives?
+ What is the average age for starting menopause in your family?
+ What treatments have they used?

Lifestyle Habits

+ Do you smoke?
+ How stressful is your life?
+ Are you satisfied with your career?
+ How well do you manage your weight?

Medications

+ What medications are you taking? Your doctor needs to know what you are taking to avoid any drug interactions.
+ What kind of complementary medicine do you practice? Complementary and natural substances can also interact with your medications.

ASSESS YOUR LEVEL OF FITNESS WITH MEDICAL TESTS

+ **Cholesterol level**: normal is 200 or less. There are two kinds of cholesterol. Total cholesterol is a combination of both the good and bad cholesterol. High cholesterol causes plaque to build up inside the walls of your blood vessels and increases the risk of heart disease.
+ **Follicle Stimulating Hormone**: assesses whether you are still producing eggs and is a good indicator of whether you have started menopause.

- **Sonogram:** takes pictures of reproductive organs and shows fibroids, etc.
- **DEXA Scanner (Dual Energy X ray Absorptiometry):** tests level of bone mass or bone density for diagnosing osteoporosis.
- **Thyroid:** problems with your thyroid cause symptoms similar to menopause.
- **Mammogram:** detects microscopic breast cancer cells.
- **Blood Pressure:** normal is 120/80. The higher number represents systolic blood pressure, the pressure when the heart is contracting. The lower number represents diastolic pressure, the pressure when the heart is relaxing. When these numbers are above 140/90, it means your heart has to work too hard.
- **Body Fat Percentage:** women between ages forty to fifty-five tend to have a percentage that is 10–15 percent higher than younger women. Body fat of 22 percent to 25 percent is good.

> **"Wellness is an active process of becoming aware of and making choices toward a more successful existence."**
>
> *—National Institute of Wellness*

Get it together

Menopause is a time when you need to make informed choices about your health care and the quality of your life. Once you have the best information available, you are in a better position to take the next step to work closely with your health care provider.

CHAPTER 4

Establish a Partnership with Your Doctor

It's quite common for African-Americans to distrust the medical establishment, but I knew I needed to get it together and make an attempt to work closely with a doctor of my choice. There were many reasons why I had not been inclined to trust my physicians. We all have a story to tell. I have been examined by medical experts who did not take time to help me relax or to talk with me about how I felt. Consequently, I have kept my doctors at a distance for most of my life. Going through menopause helped me realize the error of my ways. I encourage you to develop a collaborative agreement with a physician or caregiver right away.

The changes I faced during menopause made this relationship more important. This transition has involved a learning curve where I recognized the value of consulting with a knowledgeable and compassionate specialist. I have always preferred to wait until I was in crisis before asking for help. Doing this did not serve me well during menopause. I decided to take charge of my health by sharing all the information I had gathered about menopause with my doctor. When her initial response was positive, it turned the tide for me. I began to develop a collaborative relationship with her and she appreciated my input, my insight, and my intuition about my body.

The synergy that my doctor and I established helped me prepare for getting well. I let go of the negative conditioning that caused me to settle for less than I deserved. Being angry about how Blacks have been treated by the health care establishment in the past served no purpose unless I was prepared to use it to channel my anger in a positive manner. I changed my behavior and beliefs, and my doctor responded with her typical kindness and caring. We communicated well, and, lo and behold, I became accountable for my health.

I want to share with you how I found the perfect doctor for me. As I started to prepare myself for surgery, I began to ask women for referrals. My good friend Jacque referred me to Dr. Barbara Levy. She had read about Barbara in local newspapers and heard good comments about her from lots of her clients. Jacque is a manicurist in a very popular salon and day spa. She talks to women all day and was in an excellent position to hear their concerns. Her clients raved about Barbara Levy. Jacque had delayed asking for an appointment because she wasn't ready. She said, "Dr. Levy is the best, but you have to be ready to take charge of your health when you start working with her."

Dr. Levy's philosophy is to treat women as whole people. She establishes a collaborative agreement with each patient. She lets you know that you are in good hands and she doesn't hesitate to tell you what you need to do for yourself in order for healing to occur. We can't develop an "attitude" if we feel overwhelmed and confused. Often there is disconnection between how we feel and how our doctors tell us we should feel. This can make us feel inadequate.

As we started discussing my condition, her style was very methodical but engaging. I described my symptoms and menstrual irregularities in detail, and told her that I had been diagnosed with fibroid tumors, a condition common to many African-American women in midlife. I told her I had hoped to get through menopause without surgery because I heard that fibroids shrink during menopause. I shared information about Black women's health that I had learned from reading the Black Women's Health Project Newsletter.

She wanted to know everything I knew about my family medical and menopausal history. We also discussed my cultural beliefs about menopause and my beliefs that most Black women were in denial about the impact of this turning point on their lives. We briefly discussed the negative views of menopause in our society.

She told me about her previous experience with women with my problems and the different methods she used to avoid an incision whenever possible. She talked about using noninvasive procedures and explained all the reasons that might lead her to recommend surgery. I learned a lot from her that day.

No one else had explained to me the consequences of endometriosis, a condition where uterine tissue grows outside the uterus and can grow on other organs like the bladder and intestines, leading to other complications. Since my endometriosis was never painful, I thought it wasn't a serious condition. I really liked and respected her. She earned my trust because she valued me and addressed my concerns. She offered to use my old sonogram so I wouldn't have to go through the procedure again. I told her that I would prefer to do it again so we could start fresh on everything.

I felt that I knew her as a doctor and as a person at the end of my first appointment. This meeting was very therapeutic for me. I am a psychologist and a great communicator. I recognize when a person has extraordinary communication skills and the ability to make people feel nurtured.

I transferred some of my load to her competent shoulders that day, and I finally felt like I had a medical partner with the knowledge and compassion to help me on this journey. She was open to my thoughts and feelings and did not become uptight when I questioned her recommendations. I have to admit that I wasn't easy to work with during that first meeting because I was trying so hard to minimize my problems. I wanted there to be an easy solution.

During my pelvic exam, she was very thorough but gentle and explained everything she saw. I felt comfortable enough to ask questions about simple things like the acne that had developed on my chest. She said that because I was working out more, my perspiration was probably causing that problem.

Her way of telling me that I had some serious problems was to say something was going on with my ovaries and she wanted to see my next sonogram as soon as possible.

On our second appointment, she was warm but spoke in a somber manner. She recommended surgery as soon as possible because there were large fibroid tumors and endometriosis covering my ovaries, fallopian tubes, and uterus. Surgery was necessary in order to be sure my ovaries were not cancerous. She was firm about what needed to be done. She listened when I told her I knew I didn't have cancer because I am too in touch with my body to have a serious illness without any awareness. She said, "I don't think you have cancer either, but I'm going to be in a stew about it until we find out for sure."

In a manner-of-fact way, she began talking about possible dates for surgery and told me what to expect. By this time I was close to crying. I knew that I couldn't postpone taking action any longer. I was stunned, but I began to ask her a lot of questions. The more we talked about the specifics of surgery and menopause, the easier it became for me to get a grip on my emotions. My "strong Black woman" mode kicked in and I began telling myself that I was going to face this challenge with courage. Her final statement to me that day was, "We are going to get you well." It was several weeks after my surgery that she told me more detail about the serious complications I could have faced if the endometriosis had began to spread to my intestines and bladder. She said later she felt she had to walk a fine line to keep from scaring me, but that she had to make sure I understood that surgery was imperative.

PREPARING FOR MY HYSTERECTOMY

Dr. Levy walked me through the process step by step. She explained it would take two to three hours, and described the recovery process. She asked me to take a lot of vitamin C to help in the healing process.

She assured me that I wouldn't be sick, but that I would go into menopause immediately. I didn't really understand the significance of surgical menopause at the moment, but I knew I needed to start reading up on it. I was motivated to gather as much information as possible and to talk with my friends and family about their experiences so I would know what to expect.

I confided that I was against taking estrogen. I had been misinformed and had developed some strong opinions about hormone replacement therapy. She explained that it would be too traumatic to my system to go without estrogen because she would have to remove my ovaries. This meant she would have to put a low-dosage estrogen patch on my abdomen while I was in the recovery room. We discussed the pros and cons of hormone replacement therapy, and she gave me some medical articles to read. She asked me to try to be open-minded.

My husband and I had scheduled a trip to Trinidad for Carnival in early February. We had been looking forward to this vacation for more than a year. I asked her if she felt that I would be ready to travel four and a half weeks after my surgery. She told me that I would be able to do so but I should plan on resting several hours each day and that I wouldn't be able to participate in the dancing.

As we talked about what would happen after the surgery, she asked about my family situation and if I would have someone to stay with me. I explained that my husband is a professional speaker and would have to leave town five days after my surgery. I told her that I would call my mother to come from Detroit to be with me. Although I was still scared, I started to focus on the quality of my self-talk. I began boosting myself by saying, "I have what it takes to make a fast recovery." Actually, I said "miraculous recovery," not wanting to limit myself.

Over the next few days, I called my family and close friends and told them that I was ready to be operated on. I tried to talk to my husband, Lester, again about some of the psychological ramifications. I knew he thought that once I recovered from the surgery, everything would be the same. I knew differently.

During our pre-op appointment, Dr. Levy shared a little history with Lester about women's health, helped him to understand that menopause is not an illness, and talked about how menopause used to come toward the end of a woman's life before our life span increased. They discussed the care and support I would need during recovery. Lester felt comfortable talking with her and she encouraged him to discuss his concerns. Of course, he was terrified and didn't want to admit it. He's a typical male and wanted to have minimal discussion of the gory details.

I was reassured by her attention to detail and I felt I could rely on her foresight to get me ready. She asked several questions (such as whether motion sickness was a problem for me) and other things that would help her prepare my medications and other needs. She told me that she didn't want me to feel any pain. I felt relieved because I was really afraid of being in a lot of pain. She told me she would inject painkillers in my incision while I was still "out" to minimize the pain. I felt that she was doing everything in her power to make sure that I was comfortable. She gave me a prescription that day so I could have pain medication at my home when I returned from the hospital.

She also told me that I could go home twenty-four hours after surgery if I wished. This meant a lot to me. Dr. Levy believes that you heal better at home. She made sure I understood that I had to have a normal temperature, have no complications, and be able to take a shower by myself. I had to be able to eat at least light foods, and my pain had to be controlled by the medications she had given me to use at home. She offered to give me a sleeping pill the night before surgery. She cared as much about my feelings as she did about my medical condition.

Prior to my surgery, she talked to me outside the operating room. She wanted to know if I was warm enough and if I had any questions. I told her I was ready. I had been preparing myself mentally with affirmations, positive imagery, and self-talk. One of the most important things she did was to touch me on my shoulder and arm. As I was lying there in that bed waiting to be wheeled into the operating room, that touch meant everything. My husband was outside and couldn't come in, and everyone was very pleasant, but I had begun to feel dehumanized by the technology and all the machines around me and really needed to have my humanity reaffirmed.

That evening, when Dr. Levy came to see me, I was sitting up and feeling great. She said, "You look good." She made me feel even better. She told me I had lost a lot of blood, and seemed to have bounced back from that loss quickly. I was up walking three hours after I got out of recovery and was proud of my resiliency. She told me she would make sure that I got my medication promptly.

During my first follow-up visit, Dr. Levy and I continued strengthening our partnership. She shared information with me about every aspect of my operation. I realized that my condition was worse than what she had imagined even after years of performing this type of surgery. She had asked another surgeon to assist her because she anticipated the difficulty of the procedure, and said she was really tired when she got home that night.

About two weeks after my surgery, I asked her opinion about going to Boston to see my goddaughter, Stephanie. As was my nature, I was pushing the limit. She said traveling to Boston so soon and then going on to Trinidad two weeks later would be too tiring. She didn't hesitate to tell me I was pushing too much.

As we talked more about menopause, I told her I felt compelled to write a book on coping with menopause for African-American women. She had given me a small booklet she had written as part of her surgery package that was crystal clear in explaining every aspect of the surgery and recovery. I had read it several times, but thought a book from my perspective on what I have learned in combination with her medical expertise could be valuable, educational, and inspiring for women of color.

I offer the following tips to help African-American women establish a partnership with a primary caregiver:

Find someone highly recommended by others. Talk to other women and contact your local women's health organizations. Don't be afraid to shop around. We shop around before making decisions about houses, jobs, and other major things in our lives. Finding a good doctor is of major importance.

Make sure you feel comfortable talking with your doctor. Find someone who allows you to express your feelings and concerns. Try talking to your doctor about what's on your mind and just check out the response. If at first he or she doesn't respond to your concerns, let him or her know how you feel. Give him or her more than one chance, and if the doctor fails you again, you should consider finding someone else.

Select someone who will take the time to listen. Even when you are misinformed, like I was about hormone replacement therapy, it is important to have someone who will help you understand that you need to gather more information, someone who cares about your issues and makes every effort to see you in the full context of who you are.

Learn your doctor's health care philosophy. It was important to me that Dr. Levy shared with me her philosophy about health care. She believes in treating the whole woman and is focused on healing as opposed to just curing symptoms.

Find someone who is qualified and competent. Make sure they have a lot of experience treating women with your condition. Check credentials. Have they been certified in their area of specialty by the appropriate board, such as the American College of Obstetrics and Gynecology? How many patients has the doctor cared for who had the particular problem you have?

Find someone you like and respect. Although your doctor is the expert on women's health, you are the expert on how you feel. When Dr. Levy and I talk, it's an easy give-and-take. Our intuition about our bodies is important, and we should be encouraged to talk about our theories on what's going on with us. I like talking with someone who values what I have to say and who validates my feelings. I have attended several events and programs sponsored by Dr. Levy's women's center and have talked with lots of her patients. We all experience her the same way.

Don't settle for a doctor who is detached. Find someone who loves what they are doing. When people are doing what they love, they put so much more care and enthusiasm into each activity. I believe that Dr. Levy is a true healer who is dedicated to helping each woman have the best quality of life possible. Her values shine through. It is clear that she is doing exactly what she was meant to do.

Keep a journal of your health care. Write about your feelings, thoughts, and questions, and take this journal with you to your appointments to keep you focused. Keep a calendar of your symptoms so that you will be able to accurately discuss their duration and frequency.

Talk about your feelings even when you are confused. Don't expect your doctor to be a mind reader. Do not deny when something is wrong. After I got back from my trip to Trinidad, I was feeling strange. This was about six to eight weeks after my surgery. My menopause was full-blown and a part of me didn't want to face it. I was not sleeping, but kept rationalizing that menopause was a major adjustment and that it would get better.

As I mentioned before, I called Dr. Levy's office for an appointment. I was dressed up in a designer suit and everyone complimented me on how great I looked. I was thinking, "If I look this good, nothing could really be wrong with me." "Strutting our stuff" even when we feel lousy is something that we African-American women do well. This visit was an opportunity for me to mention that I felt something wasn't right, but I didn't take advantage of it. It was like I wanted her to know what was happening inside without any input from me. I think a part of me just wanted to continue being her star patient who was skating easily through everything. I didn't want to be in menopause and wasn't prepared to admit I was floundering.

I was using an estrogen skin patch, a small circular device similar to a Band-Aid, as described in chapter 2. Estrogen skin patches are placed on the abdomen and release tiny amounts of estrogen continuously. Mine was not effective in alleviating most of my symptoms. I dropped the ball and stopped communicating with Dr. Levy, and did not allow her to help me figure out what was happening. I wanted everything to be fine and pretended that it was. I felt like she did her part with the surgery, and it was up to me to do my part conquering menopause.

Talk about your symptoms and ask for help. A couple of weeks later, I called Dr. Levy's office and was told she was on her way to Geneva, Switzerland. I panicked. Knowing she was going to be out of touch for three weeks made me finally admit that I couldn't sleep and was experiencing mood swings and lack of concentration. I normally read four to five hours per day, but found that I couldn't read for more than a few minutes. I also couldn't finish projects. I wasn't functioning properly and my level of productivity was very low. Dr. Levy told me that I needed an estradiol blood test right away to assess my estrogen level and to determine the level of estrogen my body was absorbing from the patch. I rushed to the lab at my family doctor's office, which was only ten minutes away, and had it sent to her office.

The next day the results came back and were faxed to her. My estrogen blood level was well over 100 and in the normal range. There was no time to see her before she left so I told her I was going to see my family doctor while she was away. This decision resulted in a totally different treatment plan. My family doctor's first action was to increase the dosage of my patch to see if it helped me. It did not help me feel better and he refused to increase it a second time.

After three visits, he couldn't figure out what the problem was, but decided to put me on Premarin, an estrogen pill that comes in several different dosages and treats menopausal symptoms like hot flashes, night sweats, and insomnia. He refused to increase the dosage when I didn't get better. I was still suffering, but he told me trying to live symptom-free was unreasonable. Needless to say, I stopped seeing him. I was not willing to accept his philosophy that wanting to feel good again and wanting to be able to sleep through the night was not reasonable.

Use a variety of wellness strategies. Natural remedies are complementary to traditional allopathic medicine. When you have a serious hormonal deprivation, the natural products may not be enough. There is a strong trend toward using natural remedies, but we may be going too far in that direction. I believe the best results will come from using several types of medicine tailored to your specific situation.

Don't give up if you go to someone who can't help you. Meeting with my family doctor proved frustrating because it was obvious he did not know what treatment I should have. He tried to make me less anxious by cracking jokes, but I was too tired to respond. I asked to try a higher level of estrogen, but he said it wasn't necessary. He referred me to a sleep-disorder clinic, where I was evaluated and learned helpful tips about developing good sleep habits. But I still wasn't sleeping well. My sleep specialist finally gave me sleeping pills so I could get some rest. She cautioned me about taking them more than two to three nights per week because they were not going to solve my problem in the long run.

Follow the beliefs of our culture. African-American people have a history of using shamans and healers. We know intuitively that belief in the healer plays a role in the healing process. Unfortunately, our negative experiences with the way we are treated in America have led us to expect the worst. We have to get over this and be willing believe that the right doctor is out there.

Finally, months later, I sent Dr. Levy a letter suggesting that my inability to sleep was due to a hormonal imbalance and that I had not been able to cure it with natural remedies, and that the Premarin that my family doctor prescribed didn't appear to be working, either. She told me that she suspected my problems were related to a lack of estrogen because nothing was different in my life except that she had removed my ovaries.

She called me in immediately for several tests, all of which were normal. She told me that she felt that I had suffered too long in my efforts to use complementary medicine. I had to agree. She said, "We are going to break this pattern now." She increased my estrogen from .625 to 1.25 for two weeks, and then I tried a lower dosage of .9 for two weeks. I recorded how long I slept and the quality of sleep I experienced.

Eight hours after I took the first Premarin 1.25 sample that she gave me, I felt drowsy for the first time in months. It was a wonderful feeling. My entire life began to feel normal again. I could concentrate, I was in control of my mood, and I just felt "right" in my skin. It was so simple. Increasing my estrogen gave me back the gift of sleeping, and I will never take the act of sleeping for granted again.

Things to consider

♦ How much experience has your health care provider had working with women in menopause?
♦ What is your doctor's philosophy about wellness?
♦ How much time do you get to talk with him or her?
♦ Does your doctor respond well when you ask questions?
♦ Do you feel comfortable discussing your feelings with this person?
♦ Is your doctor accredited or certified by the medical board in his or her area of expertise?
♦ What is the quality of referrals he or she gives you?

Before going on a search for a new doctor, I took the time to review all of my previous contacts with health care providers. I listed the things that I didn't like. This helped me to clearly define what I wanted. Think about what you want from your health care provider, things like is he or she:

♦ A good listener?
♦ A person with whom you feel comfortable discussing your problems?
♦ A practitioner who respects your feelings?
♦ Someone who keeps up with the latest techniques and controversial issues on women's health?
♦ Someone who explains things clearly and still doesn't mind when you have trouble understanding them?

Doc Talk — Dr. Carolle Jean-Murat

Dr. Carolle Jean-Murat is an African-American gynecologist and author of *Menopause Made Easy.* She is the medical director of the Wellness Center for Midlife Women at Alvarado Hospital in San Diego, and has the following message for African-American women: "When an illness is diagnosed early, treatment has the greatest potential for resulting in a cure. The majority of diseases, including cancer, can be successfully treated if they're discovered early. That is why prevention and early detection is preferable."

Dr. Carolle, as she is affectionately known, encourages African-American women to take charge of their health by getting regular checkups and by paying attention to their bodies. She suggests that we give up negative habits that interfere with our health and reminds us that being healthy and having a good relationship with our primary caregiver is a matter of choice. We all need someone who cares and is willing to work with us, but we must do our part to gain knowledge and be proactive. Interviewing Dr. Carolle was inspirational. I imagine her patients begin to feel better the minute they see her.

Doc Talk — Dr. Barbara Levy

Dr. Levy defines her philosophy about patient care:
- ◆ Approach patients as unique individuals.
- ◆ Help patients transcend their anxiety and fear about their physical symptoms so true healing can take place.
- ◆ Help the patient move from a victim mentality to seeing herself as a partner in her own recovery.
- ◆ Help the patient begin to believe her symptoms are real and that her physician cares enough about her to work with her to improve the quality of her life.
- ◆ Beginning to love and care for oneself is an essential step in the process of recovery.

◆ Acceptance of the holistic approach is crucial to success.
◆ Maximize the quality of life and eliminate suffering, not necessarily to cure disease.

Ask Dr. Levy

Q: What type of info should a woman gather and take in for her first appointment when she starts to have concerns about menopause?

A: The most important thing you can do is to keep a calendar or diary in which you record your menstrual cycles and separately list your symptoms and your periods because the symptoms are not always related to the periods. A physician can make note of migraine-headache patterns, patterns of breast tenderness, and patterns of irritability and decide when they are related to your menstrual cycle. Remember, there are lots of other things that happen to women in the same age group, such as thyroid disease, and there are lots of things a physician needs to think about. Reliable and solid diary information is really important. For instance, you can note whether sleep disturbances, hot flashes, and night sweats occur just before a period. Do they occur all month long? What's really happening with the flow pattern? What's happening with sexuality? All those things are very helpful in diagnosing your problem.

Q: What defines a good doctor–patient relationship from your point of view?

A: I don't think there's anything that defines it better than a give-and-take relationship, where the woman feels heard, feels validated, and feels that her concerns have been listened to. And the physician feels that the woman is respecting her point of view. We may not always agree, but we can at least agree to disagree. I don't necessarily buy into everything that a woman believes for herself. It's my job to explain to her why I don't believe in something. I have to have the respect for the patient who says, "You do what you feel like you need to because it's your body." But don't expect me to prescribe it.

ASKING FOR HELP

Sometimes it is easier for me to express my feelings by writing things down. As I began to realize that some of my symptoms were getting out of control, I wrote the following letter to Dr. Levy asking for help. I tried to give her as much information as possible and I tried to describe my feelings clearly. I had not spoken to her about my health in six months at the time this letter was written.

Dr. Levy:

I am experiencing severe insomnia, which began in March when I finished my pain medication. Since my last appointment with you, I have consulted my family doctor as well as Dr. Moen at the Sleep Disorder Clinic. Dr. Moen prescribed Ambien, a sleeping pill. I try not to take it more than 2–3 nights per week. She also advised me to develop a sleep ritual two hours before bedtime, and had me keep a sleep journal.

I have been working hard to educate myself about menopausal conditions and have tried to master this problem on my own because I thought some discomfort and adjustment was inevitable. But after all this time, it seems clear to me that this is a serious condition and I don't know what to do.

I'd like to get your feedback and find out what you recommend as treatment at this point. I'm operating on very little sleep and it is affecting my entire life.

Sincerely,
Carolyn Scott Brown

The following is a letter written by a friend of mine. She was having a lot of problems with menopause when I first met her and she eventually traveled to Seattle to have a consultation with Dr. Levy. She sent this letter to Oprah and appeared on her show titled "The Big M":

Dear Oprah:

I am a forty-five-year-old divorcee with two grown daughters. Five years ago, I underwent a hysterectomy and my life derailed as I was thrown into early menopause. Since that time, I have gained at least sixty pounds and four to five dress sizes. That alone has been a blow to my ego—after all, I was a college queen and tagged the lady with the million dollar walk! No matter how much I try to convince myself that it is the person inside that counts, I know as a public-relations practitioner that first impressions are very important. (I could almost hear them saying, if she lets her body go like that, how can I trust her with my business?)

I was so skinny as a teen and into young adulthood that I often prayed for a big behind. Regretfully, menopause has given me that and more, especially thighs, and arms that are too fat and a gut that makes me look like I am pregnant. Not only has menopause attacked me physically, but also emotionally and professionally. As owner of a public-relations firm, I have had to make many presentations—sometimes in the midst of a presentation, I have to excuse myself or struggle through looking crazed as my body betrays me by becoming dripping wet from head to toe: $65 hairstyle gone, makeup rolling down my face with big drops of perspiration, blouse wet, suit wet, feet swashing, and all the estrogen, vitamins, ice water, and visualization therapy worth nothing when I need them most. The hot flashes worked on my confidence so much that I began to limit my presentations and projects to ones that I could get by on with limited public appearances. This was financially painful.

Mood swings got so bad that on occasion I became impatient with clients, even hanging up on one of my biggest and most faithful clients. That was my moment of reckoning—me, a person who teaches customer relations, losing her cool.

Furthermore, since the hysterectomy, my energy level has changed. I used to run five miles a day, sometimes uphill, however, now it is a struggle for me to walk five miles a day—making my million-dollar walk something of a fifty-cent slow drag. I was once considered super-woman, now those who call me at home ask "Are you still in bed"? Yes, but I didn't sleep so well last night—I woke up in sweats and hot flashes—is usually my silent answer.

It seems now, as I am older and supposedly smarter, that I have little control over my body. I try low-level estrogen and I still get hot flashes, or "power surges," as some feminists might say. I up the dosage and I get fibrocystic tender breast—which is scary, since I am at high risk for breast cancer. I am at a crossroads trying to manage my health. Will I ever return to my normal size? Please, don't tell me that it's how I eat and exercise—that hasn't worked yet. There must be more to the phenomena called menopause. Am I stuck on hormones for life? Please tell me that patience, understanding, laughter, basketball, tennis, and at least size eleven dresses will return to my life. I have faith that you either know the answer or know somebody who has the real answer to the mysteries of menopause. Will there be a time when my loved ones can stop asking "Did you take your pill this morning"?

Today my friend reports she is feeling much better. Her estrogen replacement therapy is effective and her flashes are under control. She feels she is doing a better job coping with her moods and has started several new projects. Losing weight and exercising contributes to her feelings of taking charge. She hopes to establish a relationship with a physician in her area, but will continue to work with Dr. Levy in the meantime.

This letter is a very good description of her thoughts, feelings, expectations, and the medical facts about her condition. It matches the advice of Alan N. Schwartz, M.D., Richard Jimenez, Tracy Myers, M.H.A., and Andrew Solomon, M.D. in *Getting the Best From Your Doctor*. They developed a technique called HOPE: Historical Facts, Opinions and Feelings, Personal Fears, Expectations, and Requests.

MENOPAUSE CALL TO ACTION

♦ Find a caregiver willing to work with you in a caring manner.
♦ Improve your active listening skills and communication skills so you can express your feelings effectively.
♦ Be open-minded to the information given to you about menopause.
♦ Work on your relationship with your primary caregiver.
♦ Make a commitment to increasing your level of trust.

CHAPTER 5

Get a Grip on Those Moods

African-American women are known for having the blues. It's part of our mystique and often seen as a legacy from our ancestors. I define the blues as being in a bad mood that could be caused by recent events or an accumulation of events from our past. The blues can lead to depression. Learning to recognize the signs and symptoms of when the blues cross over into depression is the first step to greater awareness. This awareness forces us to attend to our emotional barometer.

However, the topic of mood disorders and depression is a big subject and often confusing. We have been told midlife transition and depression are based on stereotypes of older women who are out of control. In reality, our emotions can swing from moodiness and feeling the blues to mild depression/stress overload, and from there to chronic depression. You may experience all of these, some of them, or none at all. Sometimes they will be related to the same circumstances or events and sometimes they won't. Taking estrogen will help to some degree for some of us. Others may need an antidepressant. But when the cause is related to the psychological issues of midlife, such as fear of aging, stress, loss of identity, and conflicting roles, we will need to utilize other strategies. Determining where we are on this continuum is paramount.

Let us begin by discussing information that will help you take a look at your moods and determine for yourself where you are on this continuum. I'm sure you can pinpoint a time in your life when you felt moody and frustrated because your life was out of control and you were agitated about problems that may have seemed insurmountable at the time. You recognized that this was a temporary state and eventually you solved your problems and moved on. At midlife, some of us are vulnerable to feeling low due to difficulties in handling the complexity of our lives and not necessarily because of menopause per se, although the physical changes during perimenopause and menopause may feel like the last straw.

Perhaps you felt the following:
♦ An inability to bounce back from defeats and disappointment
♦ Anger at family members, friends, and associates because they demanded too much of your time
♦ An inability to make decisions and put your life in perspective
♦ Overwhelmed by your daily responsibilities

"Contemporary blues" is an expression describing the trials and tribulations I face as a Black woman leading an independent life. The causes range from bad choices and bad relationships to career-related stresses and family problems. It is an expression for a temporary state that will pass or be resolved. Depression is a much more serious condition.

WHAT IS DEPRESSION?

Depression is a serious illness often described as a period of low moods that last for more than two weeks. Different people describe depression and other mood disorders as a feeling of deep sadness, hopelessness, fatigue, and isolation. These mood disorders are influenced by many factors, including stress, low self-esteem, culture shock, hormonal flux, negative attitudes, negative self-talk, family history, and traumatic life events. Even though they might be experiencing a serious mood disorder, African-American women may have difficulty pinpointing the cause because we are so good at rationalizing how we feel. We put our feelings away in a box to be dealt with later. Sometimes "later" never comes. We don't take the time to analyze what's going on. Maybe you realize you're feeling bad but just put on a happy face, as Dr. Levy tells me I was prone to doing at the beginning of my transition.

The depression caused by biological factors relates to chemical messengers in the brain called neurotransmitters. Their function is to facilitate communication between brain cells. A deficiency of these neurotransmitters causes our nerves to function improperly. This type of mood disorder/depression is effectively treated by antidepressants that help the brain hold on to serotonin, a mood lifter. When serotonin levels are adequate, they fill in the spaces around the nerves and enhance mood. Depression can also be caused by other factors, including an underactive thyroid or vitamin and mineral deficiencies. Your doctor can help you determine if you have a condition related to these factors.

For some of us, depression is related to psychological issues and is triggered when we are stressed out, angry, and frustrated. I am convinced that when many of us African-American women succumb to stress, it is due to a lot of unresolved psychological pain. Notice I use the word "succumb," because we don't give into our symptoms easily.

There is a wide variety of symptoms common to depression. Take a moment and select the symptoms that apply to you.

Symptoms of depression
♦ Lack of self-confidence
♦ Inability to feel joy or experience pleasure

- Low energy, low sex drive
- Changes in sleep patterns
- Difficulty in concentrating/memory
- Feelings of isolation
- Persistent feelings that everything is a struggle
- Feelings of hopelessness
- Extreme changes in appetite
- Thoughts of suicide

Did you know...

Did you know approximately 25 percent of all African-American women suffer from some form of depression? The other 75 percent are dealing with their issues as best they can and may be prone to feeling the blues without really needing treatment. But their coping mechanisms may not always be appropriate.

Did you know only 30 percent of women who suffer from depression ever ask for help?

Did you know many African-American women cope with their moods through faith and prayer?

Did you know the World Health Organization ranks depression in the top five of the world's most devastating illnesses?

Did you know women are most vulnerable to depression during times of great hormonal flux—teenage years, post-partum, and just prior to menopause?

WHAT HAVE WE BEEN TAUGHT ABOUT DEPRESSION?

We know our ancestors experienced and overcame a great deal of pain. They treated menopause as a passing phase without taking much time to dwell on how it impacted their lives because life was based on hard work and trying to be safe in an unsafe environment. As the old saying goes, "They just kept on keeping on." They overcame crisis situations because of a strong will to live. They were stoic and they persevered. But here we are, three or four hundred years later, often attempting to use obsolete coping skills passed down through generations. These stories and legends are based on old belief systems and cultural conditioning. Our life today is very different and the stresses we deal with are just as powerful, but require us to develop different coping strategies. Although racism and sexism are alive and well in this country, it does not serve us well to deal with it in the same manner as our grandmothers did. We also have to learn to cope differently with relationship problems and work-related problems, as well as the usual daily racial assaults on our psyche. Different coping strategies will be covered later in this chapter.

If your home training was anything like mine, you were raised to expect hardship in life and taught to be courageous and independent. We were told we would triumph over every challenge, those that are real and those that are self-imposed by the sometimes ridiculously high standards we set or allow others to set for us. In our book of life, failure is never an option! Our happiness has always been tied to overachieving, and our mindset is: "If attaining this goal makes me happy, fine, but if it doesn't I will persist and be successful anyway." A lack of happiness and joy never stopped us from doing anything. We are a generation of women of color who have made up our minds to have the best of everything. But we must look at the cost to our emotional health. Taking time to live life more consciously and replenish our inner reserves will help lower the cost.

Intellectually, you and I understand that nothing is more basic to our well-being at midlife than making sure we have learned the necessary life lessons on how to have peace of mind and a well-balanced lifestyle. We have to learn to handle mood swings, anxiety, stress, and mood disorders by being kinder to ourselves and more in touch with our feelings. In your early stages of menopause, don't ignore your low moods, lack of confidence, and crisis of esteem, as I did. Avoid trying to regain control by forcing things to work your way or by repressing your feelings. We have been there, done that all of our lives. Don't keep pushing to maintain your regular pace; take a little time to ease into midlife.

One step I took was to try my usual methods of self-care, such as engaging in positive self-talk, reading everything I could get my hands on, listening to music, and talking to girlfriends about how I was feeling. There were times when I resorted to overeating to comfort myself, even though I knew it was self-destructive behavior.

Sometimes we go to our families for help or encouragement when we are facing a challenge. This isn't always a good idea, because talking to them may not help because of the way they view us. Our parents feel such a sense of pride about our accomplishments and see us as being so strong and self-sufficient that they are uncomfortable with seeing us struggle. Perhaps they feel inadequate about advising us because our lives appear to be quite different and our challenges are so easy from their point of view. They don't get it. Often when I shared my problems, my parents told me about how they overcame everything through sheer determination, hard work, and prayer. Although it wasn't their intention, these discussions made me feel worse for complaining.

My mother and I talked almost daily in the beginning of my journey into menopause. But she was so shocked at how bad I was feeling, there were times when she was speechless, which is saying a lot. Often she could do nothing but listen. Sometimes having someone listen to me vent helped, but at other times it only reinforced my low mood. I needed solutions but didn't know where I could find them. I didn't want to look within. I didn't want to slow down and really think about how my psychological issues were aggravating my symptoms.

In my community, depression was seen as an indulgence. Folks felt like we didn't have time to feel bad about life. It was supposed to be hard, and all you had to do was get a good education, a good job, and raise your family. They saw increased economic and educational opportunities as a panacea for any problems.

Certainly, talking to a mental-health professional is not on the menu. It is not OK to ask a stranger for help with something like depression. I was taught that I can take care of my problems and that I have the strength to overcome all obstacles to becoming a successful person. Keeping things to myself or only sharing my feelings within a very close-knit circle of family and friends is the way I was raised. According to anthropologists, this behavior was healthy for slaves who were forced to develop a culture in this new land based on kinship patterns carried over from West Africa. Hiding our feelings is part of our African-American culture that was often dictated by necessity. In order to survive, we had to be secretive, stick together, and hide our feelings.

Today, I find myself in the position of wanting to keep my heritage intact, but I must learn how to adapt to a different lifestyle. My friends and I are always talking about how we made different choices than our mothers. For instance, in my immediate circle of friends from Brown University, only four of us are married and only two have children. All of us have innovative, demanding careers and are living lifestyles our mothers could only imagine. We are high achievers professionally, but may not be very good at maintaining personal balance and taking care of ourselves psychologically.

Were you conditioned, as I was, to feel breaking the silence and talking about personal problems to outsiders contributes to negative perceptions about our people? Were you coached to always be aware of the negative stereotypes assigned to African-Americans? I was taught to hold up my end and do my part to live a life of integrity and accomplishment. The responsibility of being a successful role model is a burden I was more than willing to carry, as I enjoyed the positive reinforcement I received for being the one who made it. Even when I was struggling with the stresses of my life, maintaining an image of being the healthy product of an effective and thriving family unit was more important than any relief to be gained by talking about my problems.

In the media, Black families are often described as dysfunctional, causing us to be overprotective of our family image and often leading us to deny the existence of problems like domestic violence, incest, substance abuse, and mental illness. We know these problems exist, but we don't talk about them. Many African-Americans were disturbed by the way incest, domestic violence, and mental illness were handled in the movie *The Color Purple*. We don't want to admit that this old baggage hanging out here still has power over our lives. It doesn't fit with our image today. The philosophy is, "Everyone gets the blues and every family has skeletons in the closet. Don't make a big deal of it." But the issue of our mental health is more than that, and now I understand the difference between the blues, a term we use to describe momentary sadness, and clinical depression.

A Historical Perspective

Historically, Black women have functioned as the workhorses of America and were required to take on unbelievable challenges while taking care of other people's children as well as their own. They were expected to carry the double load of performing hard work in the cotton fields of the South or menial labor in the factories of the North while taking an active role in the community. No one considered their emotional state of mind or what they needed to do to take care of themselves.

Black people are known for being stoic in the face of tremendous obstacles and adversity, and African-American women have always been at the head of the line. Our history builds good survival skills, but has conditioned Black women to believe that life is hard and that the world is hostile. The process of struggling to be happy and never quite reaching a state of happiness is often perceived as comfortable because it takes us to a familiar place where we know what to do. We persevere. I have friends who keep telling me our history is irrelevant. They don't see why I think it's pertinent to our lives today. Other people questioned the necessity of a book about menopause for African-American women. We are moving toward menopause in droves and our history is very relevant to our mental health at midlife. I tell them I believe we are a product of our history and we can't ignore the impact of the past while we build bridges to a better future.

My history as a strong Black woman sustains me. As I move forward, I recognize that change is inevitable and change can be painful, a pain tied to getting away from the familiar and forging a new path. Let us avoid taking on so many new battles and instead take the time to work on developing inner coping skills tailored to our midlife challenges. Fighting the battle to succeed while facing the tremendous isolation, sadness, and hopelessness of depression is a battle we can reject. There are many ways to define success, and living a well-balanced life is a good place to start.

Psychological Theories About Depression

The following message, from Susan Skog, in *Depression: What Your Body's Trying to Tell You* was a wake-up call for me:

> *We need to reclaim the ancient understanding of depression as a threshold to greater wholeness and healing. As painful as depression can be, it often is intended to be a wise and perfectly timed messenger; a sentinel warning us when something is amiss in our lives. A prophet pointing to*

the fact that our choices; lifestyles; spiritual, physical, and psychologi-
cal well-being may be seriously out of balance.

That passage touches me deep inside because I know my depression was a messenger. Since becoming depressed during menopause, I have made major changes in my lifestyle and have faced my unmet emotional and spiritual needs. I pay more attention to my body and do what is necessary for me to be healthy and well. I listen to inner cues that tell me when I am forcing myself to do too much, regardless of the reason. I take the time to work on projects and leisure-time activities that I enjoy, like drawing, yoga, and studying art. I heeded the call and looked inward to face what was happening to me on an emotional and spiritual level.

I discovered I was predisposed to developing a mood disorder. I can see now that this predisposition runs in my family, but it was never discussed until this generation. You can determine if you fit into this category by finding out how many members of your family have been depressed. I can think of several people in my family who were often sad or exhibited what we called antisocial behavior. They never wanted to be bothered. When they participated in family functions, we welcomed them, but we walked on eggshells trying to keep from upsetting them. Sometimes they disappeared for months and avoided family gatherings. I accepted them, and it did not occur to me that they were in need of medical attention. Whether I knew the trigger or cause of their mood disorder or not, I never thought of their problems as a medical condition.

In my community, it was OK for women to go a little crazy during menopause. Folks would say, "She started the change of life and hasn't been the same since." The general consensus was some women become depressed during menopause and there's nothing you can do about it. That's life. I know now that menopause doesn't cause depression or other mood disorders, it's all the baggage we carry into menopause that can act as a trigger.

According to Dr. Jonathan Zuess, author of *The Wisdom of Depression*, "Depression wells up and encompasses us for a time in a state of painful, dream saturated formlessness, but its true purpose is to provide the opportunity for healing insight, renewal, and reintegration."

This is an innovative way of looking at depression. The message is clear. If I see my mood disorder as an opportunity to grow and heal, then I will be more committed to putting the puzzle together to resolve my issues. I believe every experience in life happens for a reason, and there is a lesson to be learned. Looking at depression as part of a painful episode that I have to work through in order to learn more about who I am has helped me put it in perspective. I am not suggesting most African-American women will develop mood disorders during menopause, but for those of us who do, it will be helpful to look at various theories of how to process this experience.

In a similar vein, Dr. Mona Lisa Schultz, author of *Awakening Intuition*, says, "Depression is part of our intuitive guidance system. It is a warning bell that tells you something in your life is out of balance."

Some sisters tell me they have come to realize the underlying cause of their depression was something other than menopause. Many were faced with more than one challenge at menopause, and in hindsight realize the trials of menopause brought things out in the open, things they could no longer ignore. We can't continue to look for the easy solutions and blame everything on our hormones. Dr. Levy says some of her patients are too quick to look to hormones to fix emotional problems.

Vera's story is a perfect example. At the time of her interview with me, she was fifty-four. She zipped through perimenopause without realizing it and was well into menopause before she noticed that she was no longer having periods, was feeling warm all the time, and was tired, irritable, and frequently in a bad mood. She found it very difficult to get out of bed every morning even though she liked her job as an executive at a major advertising firm. After taking Prozac, an antidepressant, for several months, she began to function better and realized that her marriage was the cause of a great deal of her unhappiness. It took her seven years to face the reality that her husband was not the man she thought he was and he was never going to change.

Like many other women, she had been hanging in there with him. Using terminology that many Black women understand, she said, "He was just perpetuating being a man when deep down inside he was an inadequate, selfish child." She said, "He pretended to have goals until we got married and then achieved less and less and was content with just getting by." Vera began to feel better as soon as she let go of this negative and emotionally draining relationship. Today her menopause symptoms are being managed well with Pempro, a combination estrogen and progesterone pill. She's talking to her doctor about decreasing her Prozac, which she has been taking for a year, and hopes to get off of it in the next six months. She has started her own consulting business and looks forward to starting several new projects. Her son will be starting college in two years, and she is enjoying her relationship with him as he matures. She says menopause is turning out to be a great time of life for her.

> **"Our depression manifests itself differently. Instead of the classic 'vegetative signs' one expects to see—lack of interest in activities, trouble sleeping, failure to eat—depressed African-American patients often show increased activity—the proverbial 'laughing to keep from crying.'"**
> *—Thomas Parham, past president of the National Association of Black Psychologists*

DETERMINING WHAT'S GOING ON WITH US

Now that we have explored the biological and psychological causes of depression/mood disorders, let's determine for ourselves what's causing us to feel low. It is imperative that we learn as much as we can about mood disorders. These conditions affect more than one million African-American women. After reviewing the information, we must examine our assumptions and prepare to successfully cope with our unique brand of mood disorders. No matter if it is just the blues, stress, and burnout or long-term depression; wherever we are on the continuum, help is available. It's become clear to me it is not a case of menopause causing depression. Instead, it is a case of what we bring to this phase of life. We need to pay attention to what is going on with us before we get there.

What is it about our lives that we are responding to when we feel bad?

Maybe you are at a turning point in your life and feel overwhelmed by all your tasks and responsibilities. Your depression could be handled by getting your priorities together.

Are we experiencing the blues or a bad mood?

Are these momentary feelings that will pass in a day or two? And while we're talking about it, what about all those mood swings we've heard about?

Have you found yourself getting ticked off more often? I had tremendous mood swings during perimenopause. The biggest difference I noticed was that I became angry very fast. I would go off about little things. It was very upsetting because I knew when I was overreacting, but I couldn't control my behavior. I had no tolerance for nonsense. Needless to say, I was easily irritated with my staff, friends, and husband. As this behavior continued, I tried to break the pattern simply by controlling my self-talk. I wasn't very successful.

Once my estrogen level was increased and I was able to get more sleep, my mood swings improved. I was calmer and I felt much more in control within a few days. Let me tell you, sleep deprivation had a lot to do with my moods. I really, really need to get enough sleep to keep from being out of control. There were times I felt I should have been wearing a badge that said, "I haven't had enough sleep, so approach me at your own risk!"

When I found myself in situations that were upsetting at home or at work, I was able to think things through and respond appropriately. I had not anticipated developing mood disorders and was caught off-guard. I encourage you to be alert to the first signs of mood disorders.

CHAPTER 6

Get Rid of Old Baggage

Old baggage, repressed feelings, and too much stress impact our emotions. Sometimes it is hard to pinpoint where all this "stuff" is coming from and then generate enough energy to handle it. A review of stress management, along with suggestions for boosting self-esteem, assists us in dealing with the long-term emotional problems that may surface during the Second Half of Life.

ARE WE BOGGED DOWN BY STRESS?

We hear people talking about stress all the time, but often we don't have a clear picture of what it is and what causes stress in our lives. Not all stress is bad, and it would be impossible to totally eliminate stress. Some stress, when it is manageable, is beneficial because it gives us a competitive edge.

Medical research describes stress as the nonspecific response of the body to any demand made upon it. The key word here is "nonspecific" because it refers to any response, both positive and negative. A simpler definition coined by Dr. Hans Selye, the godfather of stress research, is that stress is the rate of the wear and tear on your life. Only you can decide how fast the rate will be.

Stress develops when we feel threatened or challenged by events or circumstances. We experience stressful feelings when we are uncertain of our ability to cope with the demands made upon us. Every time we are forced to adjust to an event, thought, or situation, it causes stress. Everyone experiences stress, but each person reacts differently to stressful situations. Sometimes we perceive something as stressful because of past experiences or our interpretation of current situations.

Answering the following questions will help you begin to gain an awareness of the role that stress is playing in your life.

WHAT SITUATIONS CAUSE STRESS FOR YOU?

Any event or situation can cause stress. Stress can also be triggered by external factors:

+ Traffic jams
+ Car trouble
+ Excessive noise
+ Daily hassles
+ Social injustices
+ Natural disasters
+ Current events
+ Deadlines at work
+ Problems with children

Stress can also be caused by internal factors (e.g., thoughts, unreasonable self-imposed expectations, low self-esteem, feelings of inadequacy, anxiety). In midlife, we can be stressed by our menopausal symptoms and the feeling that our bodies are betraying us. We can't control the world outside us, but we can control our response to it.

How Do You Respond to Events and Circumstances Beyond Your Control?

Stress can be complex and caused by a multitude of stressors. There are psychological and physiological aspects of stress. The psychological aspect concerns your feelings and emotions, resulting in feelings of anxiety and tension when something upsets you. This type of stress is often self-induced because our perception or interpretation of a situation is often biased or inaccurate. An example would be when we set unrealistic expectations, or when we see every situation as a matter of life or death. A typical response in a situation like this might be: "I'm going to do this even if it kills me!" Think back and describe a situation when you felt anxious or desperate. What were your reasons for feeling that the situation was a matter of life and death? Is feeling this way ever justified?

The symptoms related to the psychological aspect of stress are quite similar to the way we feel when we are depressed, including anxiety attacks, loss of sexual desire, irritability, and inability to make decisions.

Often we repress our feelings when we are upset, and this leads to eruptions and overreaction. We might have a tendency to explode over trivial things because we have allowed our feelings to build up. We may feel we have nowhere to turn or that everyone is against us. A feeling of powerlessness and helplessness contributes to this spiral of emotions. If we enter menopause feeling this way, it will contribute to our sense of things getting out of control.

Coping with Stress

Slow down and take time to look at what's going on. Be honest with yourself and take a hard look at every area of your life. What's out of balance? What are you doing strictly out of habit? Where are you pushing too hard?

Learn to recognize when you are having a stress response. There are three stages. The first is an alarm stage. All of the systems in the body sense a threat and go up in arms. Next, the body moves to a stage of resistance, where it mobilizes to fight the threat. This stage is often called the "fight or flight" response. In this state, we are primed to fight or run. In our world today, neither response is usually appropriate, but we are in the habit of sending the body through this alarm repeatedly. The stress response takes a tremendous toll on our bodies. The final stage is recuperation, where our body fights to return to equilibrium. We want to move to recuperation as quickly as possible to minimize the physiological and psychological wear and tear.

On a daily basis, we need to minimize the number of times we allow ourselves to get stressed. Learn to anticipate and plan for stress. Avoid taking on too many battles and getting overextended.

Control negative self-talk and affirm the results you want in each situation. Correcting your thinking skills and the way you allow your emotions to lead you to the wrong conclusions or to make false assumptions is important to this process.

AFFIRMATIONS
- I choose to handle stress in a healthy manner. I know I am in control of my perception of what's happening in my life and in charge of changing my responses.
- I am in control of the way my body and my mind respond to stress.
- My world is subject to my rational interpretation of events and circumstances in my life. I manage my psychological stress in a way that enhances my well-being and my health.

Are Your Moods Related to Low Self-Esteem and Poor Body Image at Midlife? Are You Depressed About Aging and Focusing on the Losses Tied to Midlife?

In *Sisters of the Yam*, bell hooks talks about developing "body esteem" and about how Black women need to stop obsessing about their bodies and just take care of them. There is room for improvement and we should just get on with it without negative put-downs.

Things to think about

♦ Are African-American women in this day and age more likely to become depressed during menopause?

♦ If so, is it because of our particular lifestyles, our cultural conditioning, or because of our own self-imposed pressure to always be the best?

♦ What are the stresses particular to African-American women as they age?

♦ Do we have more stress than other groups of women, and how are we coping with the stressors in our lives?

♦ How can we make better choices throughout our lives?

There have been times when I felt stressed out by the daily demands of my life. I know I am not unique in feeling this way. There have been other times when I felt incredible joy, but I began this journey feeling that menopause was another problem to solve. I don't know all the reasons why menopause triggered so many feelings for me, but I do know that it became a wake-up call for me to get more in touch with my own emotions.

Are Your Moods Related to Low Self-Esteem?

Research shows that improving self-esteem increases feelings of personal effectiveness. Nathaniel Branden, Ph.D., in *The Power of Self-Esteem*, states, "We recognize that just as a human being cannot hope to realize his or her potential without healthy self-esteem, neither can societies whose members are not valued. Self-esteem is our most important psychological resource."

Psychologists state that it is in a woman's nature to surrender to others. Our first thought is always to put others that we love first. We forget the beauty in self-love and getting our own needs met so that we can achieve our own definite aim and purpose in life. This can lead us to be victimized by love. When we let our families know what we need, they will support us.

ENHANCING POSITIVE SELF-ESTEEM
- Accept yourself.
- Affirm new beliefs with affirmations and visualization.
- Improve your feelings of self-worth through increasing accountability and credibility with yourself.
- Keep your promises to yourself.
- Change your attitudes on how you cope with your feelings.
- Become truly independent in your thinking and your behavior.

My level of personal effectiveness has increased over the years as I have worked on enhancing my self-esteem. The beginning stages of menopause worked to diminish my self-esteem until I began to feel more capable of dealing with my feelings of frustration and loss of control. I had to do some more work on my self-image. I went on a mission to eliminate negative pictures stored in my subconscious mind and to substitute positive images of myself as healthy, strong, young, vibrant, positive, harmonious, successful, and happy. This affirmation and mental image is something I have used since I read the work of Venice Bloodworth, a spiritual psychologist and author of *Key to Yourself*.

African-American women tell me they are angry. It takes hard work to channel this anger in positive ways. We have been denied equal access to the American Dream. As talented as we are, there are always ambiguous messages that imply that our best is not good enough. Redirecting that anger involves digging deep under layers of defensiveness we have to shed in order to be well-balanced and healthy.

Life Lesson

During our menopausal years, we often have a tendency to overreact to daily conflicts and minor irritations. Once you become aware that you are doing this, check your first response. Stop and clear your mind. Take a deep breath and evaluate each situation clearly. Adopt a visual reminder to help you calm down. Use a mental image of something peaceful and serene. I picture the ocean on a sunny day. I hear the waves washing up on the beach.

During menopause, there are times when you will see everything more clearly. The sun will be brighter and the colors more vibrant. These are the days when you will feel the true power and passion for life that comes from being in this wonderful time of your existence.

IS THE CAUSE FOR YOUR MOOD DISORDER PSYCHOLOGICAL, CAUSED BY UNRESOLVED CHILDHOOD TRAUMA AND FAMILY PROBLEMS?

Dr. Levy says those of us with a predisposition are more susceptible to depression during periods of hormonal change. Something acts as a trigger, our brain chemistry changes, and a serious depression starts.

I was depressed and didn't realize it. Most days I struggled to feel upbeat and happy. I felt low self-esteem and doubted myself. It was like being in quicksand, or in a fog. Then with my doctor's help, I realized I had emotional issues tied to childhood sexual abuse. I also learned there is a wealth of information available on helping women who were sexually victimized as children. This literature helped me revisit how my self-esteem was damaged and my feelings of shame of being a victim. I believe there are many

African-American women who have been forced to keep family secrets because, "Black families don't share their dirty laundry." My goal is to show you this type of thinking is detrimental to our mental well-being. We must begin to talk about what's going on with us so that we can develop strategies for dealing with our feelings. It's not necessary for me to always have all the answers or be the strong one.

I came to understand that I suppressed feelings related to prior emotional pain from childhood and the continuous struggle to be accepted in a racist and male chauvinistic society that denies my beauty, my brilliance, and my right to succeed. Suppressing these feelings is never successful for long, and they resurfaced during this most recent transition in my life. The underlying cause of my depression was not linked to a recent dramatic event, but tied to accumulated feelings that were denied, rejected, and resisted in order for me to continue functioning in a stressful world.

Depression has often been tied to feeling powerless. At midlife, if your symptoms get out of control and you find your usual coping mechanisms don't work, you may begin to feel powerless. "We must free ourselves from the burden of being strong when we feel frail," state Mitchell and Herring in *What the Blues Is All About.*

My hysterectomy was the trigger for my depression. During my annual exam two years after my surgery, I asked Dr. Levy how long I would have to continue taking an antidepressant. I explained that since my hormone levels were in check, I felt I shouldn't still be depressed. However, whenever I tried to cut down on my medication, I became depressed again within a few days.

Dr. Levy told me she suspected my depression was tied to possible child abuse. In her experience, a hysterectomy can trigger memories of pain and injury because the surgery can be experienced as a new mutilation of the sexual organs. She had to cut me along the same path of an attempted penetration. I was floored when she said this. I have always had vague memories of being molested as a child. I had shared my memories with my sister and discussed them with my therapist when I was in graduate school. I thought I had resolved my feelings about it.

During that time in my life, I had been experiencing difficulty having orgasms, and sometimes I clenched my vaginal muscles prior to penetration. Learning to meditate, using mind/body techniques like imagery and deep-breathing exercises helped me to overcome these problems. It had never occurred to me that my childhood sexual abuse was contributing to my depression at age forty-seven.

Dr. Levy explained that she could identify my problem because she knows how much I trust her, yet I always tense up whenever she examines me. Once the exam is over, I relax immediately. It was amazing to me that she suspected I had been abused. I didn't consciously hide it, but it seems clear that I have some more work to do in this area.

After my initial shock, I felt some momentary feelings of shame, which was surprising because I know that she is a compassionate person. It was like I had a terrible secret and now someone else knew about it besides my immediate family and my therapist. Then I felt like a load was lifted. I'm glad we were able to talk about it. If you're like me and have discussed memories of sexual abuse in the past and find those feelings emerging again during menopause, then it is time to face them again. If you have never been able to talk about this part of your past, then now is as good a time as any.

I cried on my way home from my annual exam, and it reminded me of crying on this same route the day I learned I had to have surgery. I have come a long way since that day, but my journey of self-discovery still continues. I shared my feelings with Lester, and then we proceeded to have one of those great weekends where you take lots of time to talk. I kept thinking of how to learn and grow from this experience.

Over the weekend, I spoke with my mom and my sister. We talked about when my sexual abuse must have happened. My sister was raped when she was almost five by my first stepfather. My mother called the police and Protective Services after finding my sister bleeding in bed. Our stepfather was arrested and my sister was placed in a foster home for six months until his trial was over and he was incarcerated. My mom said it did not occur to anyone to examine me. There was no indication I had been assaulted, but I have a memory of something huge being forced between my legs.

When I was a therapist, more than 60 percent of the women who came to see me had been abused. Every day, more and more women are talking about their experiences. I applaud them. I had discussed my situation with my husband before we were married and he was very supportive. He has always understood that I require a great deal of foreplay to help me relax. Don't be afraid to tell your partner. Give them a chance to help you overcome your fears.

I am using a book called *The Courage to Heal* to help me work through my feelings. The authors, Laura Davis and Ellen Bass, describe several things you can do to help you heal. I am following the steps that make sense to me. Make a commitment to take action right away. It will free you up to enjoy your Second Half of Life.

Why don't you:

- **Write about your experience.** I began my writing about my feelings and describing exactly what happened to me. It helped me put things in perspective.
- **Talk about your experience with your family.** I talked about what happened to me to several people, including my mom and my sisters.
- **Share your story with other women.** I share my story with other women in my menopause and motivational workshops.

♦ **Join a survivors group.** There are groups available through
community mental-health centers and family-service organizations.
Bring up this topic in your Do Menopause with An Attitude group
sessions. You may be surprised at how many other women have had
a similar experience.

What Is Causing Us to Feel Bad?

Answering this question helps us continue to assess where we are and pinpoint the underlying causes of our feelings.

Sometimes it is hard to recognize when you are depressed, especially
during times of stress and rapid change in your life. Sometimes life takes a
toll and circumstances bring us down momentarily. African-American
women are very resilient. But depression is different. It is more than a temporary setback.

Ask yourself the following questions about how you are feeling to help
you determine if it's depression or just life. What's going on in your life
right now that could be upsetting you?

Are you putting yourself under too much pressure by taking on the burdens of other people? Do you allow others to disrespect you?

When we are still operating as "superwomen" and trying to be all things
to all people, it becomes harder and harder to focus on our own emotional
needs. Also ask yourself if you are repressing your feelings when other people disrespect you or put you down. When we give others permission to
make us feel bad about ourselves and let this pattern continue over the
years, we end up getting into psychological trouble. We feel angry but
don't take action and demand respect from others, and this causes us to
have less respect for ourselves. If this anger is not dealt with, it can lead to
depression.

Are you unhappy but afraid to admit it? Have you been postponing difficult decisions because you were too busy to deal with them?

Sometimes we postpone making decisions that we know in our hearts have to be made. The longer we postpone these traumatic decisions, the harder it becomes to face them. Just thinking about it becomes very painful. The feelings we have about not facing troublesome situations in our lives develop a power of their own and bring us down.

Answering yes to the questions above could possibly indicate that life is depressing you. You may be making decisions in your personal life that you don't feel good about or allowing negative interactions with others get you down. Make a point to confront each of these issues and do what is best for you.

Put Your Life in Perspective

How would you describe yourself? What experiences have shaped you and made you the woman you are today? How can you use your particular outlook on the world to help you stay in touch with your feelings?

> **"When times get tough, rejoice in the knowledge that you are one in a long line of proud, courageous people who have a history of surviving."**
>
> —*Denise L. Stinson*

I have always seen myself as a nontraditional woman who wanted to set my own pace in the world. I wanted the freedom of not raising children, and decided at a young age that I would play the role of an indulgent "auntie" to my nieces and nephews. This has worked well for me. I guess in every family there are children who can benefit from the extra attention of a childless relative who takes a special interest in them and supplements the care they receive at home. I never felt a strong maternal instinct. This made me different from some of my friends, relatives, and associates. But it also made me realize that I had to do what felt right to me.

If you find yourself facing problems with low moods during your transition from perimenopause to menopause, take a self-assessment and become aware of opinions and beliefs that may be affecting your mental health. Think about it:

- Every woman is a product of the entire history of her sex, genes, her own past, and the negative way the world views women. We can only escape this by truly understanding how we have been locked into pleasing everyone but ourselves.
- Understanding our past history in the world will help us invent a new future.
- There are many negative perceptions of African-American women that can be limiting if we allow others to dictate to us who we are and what we are capable of achieving.
- Don't buy into stereotypes that tell us we're not smart enough, beautiful enough, or worthy of the best life has to offer.

Erroneous beliefs developed about self and our place in the world may come to the surface during midlife transition. It's possible that those of us who get depressed are still dealing with anger, self-doubt, and a lack of self-love. Perhaps we spent years doing what comes naturally to us, which is to persevere in spite of pain and adversity. Dr. Brenda Wade and Brenda Lane Richardson, authors of *What Mama Couldn't Tell Us about Love,* encourage us to think about our history and the emotional impact of slavery on our ability to love ourselves. They describe the limiting beliefs Black women have developed in order to survive and cope such as, "It's not safe for me to face my anger." They encourage each one of us to develop new beliefs about our level of self-worth.

AFRICAN-AMERICAN WOMEN MUST LEARN FROM THE PAST TO BUILD A BETTER FUTURE

Building harmony and balance involves moving out of our present comfort zone. Our comfort zone is the area in which we feel most secure and are accustomed to being. Whenever we move outside our comfort zone, we have to be prepared to experience some discomfort. This is necessary before true growth takes place. Menopause threw me out of my comfort zone. I was forced to take a look at my need to control things. I was also forced to admit that I needed help, which is something I rarely do. Most importantly, menopause got me to slow down and really evaluate what I was doing in my life. Sometimes when I get stressed out and make contact with Dr. Levy about one of our many projects, she reminds me to slow down and enjoy the sunshine. Other times she has told me that I'm trying to do too many things and that contributes to my mood swings. Sometimes it isn't depression; it's life and the choices we make.

DOC TALK—DR. BARBARA LEVY

Depression isn't sadness. It's a mood disorder. It affects our sleep, our eating habits, and our ability to feel pleasure. Women are going through a lot that has to do with women's role in our culture. We're valued for our looks. There are things we are expected to achieve that we can never achieve. It creates a sense of failure. We do not have perfect bodies, and that should be OK. We have negative self-talk, and what we tell ourselves is part of the problem. Often what we tell ourselves makes us feel inadequate.

Also, we do things that do not have an end. We do things that no one notices or thanks us for. Whatever we do is never enough. Unfortunately, we put ourselves at the bottom of the list. Women are angry. Who is there for us? Who notices when we don't feel good?

MENOPAUSE CALL TO ACTION

+ Document your moods in your menopause journal.
+ Practice controlling your self-talk.
+ Learn to manage stress and anger.
+ Discuss your feelings with your doctor and see a counselor to help you sort things out.
+ Express your feelings.
+ Begin seeing mood disorders as a sign that your life is out of balance.
+ Take time to relax and analyze what going on with you.

Ask Dr. Levy

Q: What are your patients' greatest concerns about menopause?

A: Most of the patients who come in, especially those who are younger than we would expect, are troubled by their own irritability. There is more concern about the psychological symptoms women are experiencing. A lot of it is just the role that women play in our culture. It's such a difficult time in life for women. We are not the successful, powerful executives for the most part. We're still trying to balance being mothers and wives and successful people in the workforce. There are so many people at us with so many expectations, we don't even know who we are. We don't know what we really want. We know what our bosses tell us we should be. And heaven forbid we definitely know what the media tells us we should be. So there's a lot of "dis-ease," discomfort with our measure of success personally. How we feel about ourselves compared to the measures that are out there.

My patients are women who are so frustrated with themselves that they feel unsuccessful. That feeling manifests itself in a lot of physical and anxiety-related symptoms, sleeplessness, depression, and an inability to care for oneself. Being all things to all people at all times except to ourselves. We're not very good at that.

CHAPTER 7

Celebrate Your Sexuality

As an African-American woman, I have been told I am supposed to be hot. People have been known to call us "hot chocolate." Buying into the stereotype that says all African-American women are hot makes aging and dealing with menopause more difficult. Unfortunately, there are times when we allow ourselves to adopt roles that have been assigned to us by society, even at our own expense. The stereotype of the African-American women who can "never get enough" started during slavery as a justification for raping our ancestors more than four hundred years ago and continued as a rationale for labeling all Black women as sex objects and "Jezebels" who were always "begging for it." These stereotypes still linger.

Traditional sex roles common in American society that categorize women as second-class citizens and less than equal in male/female relationships are present in African-American culture as well, but we have often enjoyed more freedom and power. Our power and opportunities came about because we were more easily accepted and less of a threat to white males in the "old southern boy network."

I am usually quite comfortable discussing my sex life with my "sistah" friends and family members. But I was reluctant to discuss these issues with a qualified professional until I met Barbara Levy. I overcame my culturally ingrained beliefs against asking her to help me solve my problems. And let me tell you, it wasn't easy! My Second Half of Life has been a time when I experienced sexual discomfort in numerous ways depending on my current menopausal symptoms. How I coped with what I expected of myself, fulfilled my husband's desires, and adjusted to my new needs in the sexual area has been key.

Asking For Help

How I approached my doctor to discuss my sexual difficulties during the first two years of my menopause journey is an interesting story. I used communication techniques perfected during my time as a therapist. First, I wrote scripts describing the problems I experienced with vaginal dryness and loss of libido. Then I practiced saying this information with minimal embarrassment and confusion. I also listed my concerns and tried to anticipate the questions that she might ask so that I could prepare carefully thought-out answers. It's often difficult for us to ask for any help with sensitive issues, and discussing sexual issues openly can be a problem for even the most self-confident person.

New Paradigms in Sexuality

The role estrogen plays in our sexuality needs to be discussed, as well as some of the myths about decreased sexual libido. I want to make it clear that nothing is absolute, and each woman's response to diminishing estrogen is different. For women of color, who have always bought into the stereotype of the "sexy mama," it can be quite frightening to wake up one day and experience difficulties in an arena where they functioned extremely well in the past.

You may need to revise your sexual self-image when you have always had a picture of yourself as being very sexy. Many African-American men and women see their sex lives as an area of ethnic pride. It's one of those culturally laden areas where we say, "At least the world recognizes that we do something well." These myths can make it more difficult for Black women to discuss sexual difficulties.

Let's take a look at sexuality and what it means to us. According to Dr. Susan Rako, sexual desire can be influenced by a multitude of factors, including situational, relational, emotional, spiritual, and physical. It's quite possible that the impact of these factors vary for women of color. Our sexual behaviors, beliefs, and patterns of intimacy are closely tied to our cultural beliefs about sexuality.

Exploring sexual issues is something we African-American women need to do. How do we see ourselves sexually? How important is it to maintain the myth that all of us are good in bed? If we begin to experience problems in this arena, what will it do our sexual self-image? Increasing our under-standing and awareness of these issues will provide psychological informa-tion we can use to facilitate an easier transition. Let's face it: being sexually proficient is part of our culture. I hate to generalize this way, because I know African-American women who were raised in environments where sexuality was portrayed as something dirty. There is some diversity in the way we perceive sexuality.

Our ability and willingness to engage in sexual fantasies and masturba-tion is also culturally determined. I am open to discussing how I pleasure myself with some of my friends who have no problem discussing their sex lives with me. But why we developed certain sexual habits, or how they can be modified or adapted during times of transition, needs to be further explored by us all.

DISCUSSING SEXUAL ISSUES WITH YOUR SEXUAL PARTNER

If and when sexual problems arise during menopause, after discussing the situation with a doctor, I encourage you to prepare to talk with your sexual partner. There are certain dynamics in many African-American relationships that may make it difficult to initiate this type of discussion. For instance, because we had more access to educational and economical opportunities than our men, our guilt about this special treatment has led us to make excuses for our men and pick up the banner of overprotection from their mothers. African-American mothers are always trying to compensate their sons for the harsh treatment of society.

As women, lovers, and sexual partners, we sometimes perpetuate the same pattern of behavior and accept the role of trying to make it up to them. We work too hard making sure they are happy in and out of bed. Being overprotective and carrying the burden for their happiness is reinforced by our feelings for all the males we love, including our fathers, brothers, uncles, and sons. It's easy to allow the fear that they will be treated like Rodney King to cause us to take too much responsibility for catering to the needs of our men in and out of bed. This can have a negative impact on our sexual relationships because it makes it difficult to ask that our needs be met. My lesbian friends tell me they don't have this problem. Apparently, it is easier for them to talk woman-to-woman about their sexual needs.

For instance, if a woman has the type of relationship where she feels comfortable asking for what she wants, it will be easier to admit that she may need special care during the beginning stages of menopause. When the sexual relationship is based primarily on pleasing her partner and adhering to inflexible roles, it may be quite difficult to raise the sexual relationship to another level. She may be reluctant to talk about her needs or express her feelings about what she wants. Saying no when she's not in the mood or letting her partner know when she needs something different, like more stroking, a different rhythm, or pressures on different points, may be difficult for her to do. If the communication lines are not open, initiating these types of discussions can be tricky. In my beginning stages of menopause, I found that I needed less friction and different movements to bring me to a certain point. I'm not sure why, but my pleasure points seem to have shifted. Take it from me, these sexual discussions can be fun. It was like I was discovering new patterns with a new partner, and that brought a sense of adventure and expectation that reminded me of our first sexual encounters more than seventeen years ago.

Dr. Levy and I believe that good sex before menopause is a predictor of good sex during and after menopause because a good sexual relationship is based on good communication. When the communication is defective, the upheaval during menopause can put a greater strain on the relationship. Even though African-American men tell me they are committed to being supportive during their wives' transitions, many admit they are fearful about how this transition will impact the ebb and flow of their sexual relationships. Whenever possible, it is good to attempt to get everything out in the open and have people air their fears.

> **"The greatest problem with communication is the illusion that it has been achieved."**
> —*George Bernard Shaw*

African-American women who are big-time caretakers will have difficulty allowing someone else to take care of them or even admitting that their sex life isn't everything they want it to be. I encourage you to think about using scripts to prepare for sexual discussions, like those I used during my time as a marriage counselor. Preparing a script to help you figure out exactly what to say is helpful. Sometimes the most difficult task is figuring out how to get started. Practice opening the discussion in several ways to find out what is most comfortable for you. Mental rehearsal is helpful as well. Think about what you want to happen and play it out in your mind.

Controlling negative self-talk is also crucial during times of transition, as self-talk impacts behavior. We can control our mind-set by focusing on the end results we want in each sexual interlude. If a negative thought or picture comes to mind, we have to substitute it with a positive picture, refusing to allow our fears to control us. The mind-set we have before sex or when we are just thinking about the next encounter is important. I prepared mentally with thoughts and pictures geared to feeling good. When my self-talk was negative because I was tired or anxious, it was harder for me to relax. I would put myself down because I wasn't responding the way I used to or because my needs had changed and I needed more time to relax and get in the mood.

Learning how to pinpoint exactly what I needed was an essential first step in facing my sexual difficulties. There were times when I found myself just wanting emotional support from my husband. At other times, I wanted to do some problem-solving where we could talk about what was happening between us, how my sexual needs had changed, and what we could do differently to increase enjoyment for both of us. When I experienced severe insomnia, I was very tired and irritable and I had a need to be comforted, but having intercourse was a very low priority. I asked that he be patient with me. I also encouraged Lester to discuss his feelings about how this journey was changing things for us. Talking really helped.

When I encountered problems due to a lack of sexual desire, another issue arose that I was not able to solve on my own. Again, I had to forego what Joan Morgan calls the "STRONGBLACKWOMEN." She writes, "I draw strength daily from the history of struggle and survival that is a Black woman's spiritual legacy. What I kicked to the curb was the years of social conditioning that told me it was my destiny to live my life as "BLACK-SUPERWOMEN Emeritus." She proclaims her retirement from this behavior pattern in her book *When Chickenheads Come Home to Roost*. This young woman was preparing to make changes in her behavior twenty years before she reached midlife.

Taking an antidepressant and having a total hysterectomy took a toll on my sex drive. Once again, after several months of delay, I shared this problem with Dr. Levy by sending her a brief email describing "one last problem I hadn't been able to solve." She called me within twenty-four hours and adjusted my medication accordingly. I am using a low-dosage testosterone cream. As close as we are, it was still difficult for me to initiate a discussion about my sexual difficulties with her. Dr. Levy and I talked later about how I delayed talking to her until I was desperate. We had already addressed my issues with vaginal dryness, and I had wanted that to be my last menopausal hurdle. It wasn't.

Life Lesson

I am through being a "STRONGBLACKWOMEN" when it comes to my health. At midlife, I recognize the value of admitting when I have a problem and need help.

Exposing and resolving the problems I have encountered since entering menopause has not been easy, but it had to be done before I could get better. Whenever I felt uncomfortable sharing my feelings with my doctor or my husband, I would discuss my situation first with my sister or with a girlfriend. Eventually, I always talked to someone. Who do you go to when you have sensitive issues to discuss? Remember, menopause is not the time to be trying to take care of everything by yourself. We need to be prepared to face this issue head-on. It is important for us to get this sex thing right and keep it together.

African-American women who are determined to excel at everything will have the most difficulty coping with sexual difficulties during menopause because we will feel more threatened when problems arise.

Some of us have a self-image in which we become the perfect mother, perfect lover, and perfect career woman. Our sexuality may be closely defined by sexual roles that say: "Black women are highly sexed." With a sexual identity tied to being "always ready," we may be devastated to find ourselves experiencing low libido, vaginal dryness, or difficulty in climaxing. But I have good news for all of us! Any problems we experience with our sexuality during menopause can be dealt with. There is no reason to lower our expectations of continuing to enjoy good sexual relations.

Each of us will need to do some self-assessment and take a hard look at our own relationships. If it is necessary to make some changes, we can determine a plan of action that will help us ask for what we need. Ask yourself the following questions:

+ How happy am I with my sexual relationship?
+ Are there sexual problems or issues I have been avoiding?
+ Do I feel comfortable talking with my partner about what I like?
+ Do I still feel sexy, sensual, and desirable?
+ What would make me feel more in tune with my body?
+ What can I do to make things right or just to add a little zest?
+ Are there medical or emotional needs that need to be confronted?

I don't mean to paint a bleak picture of sex during and after menopause. Many African-American women tell me their sex lives and sexual enjoyment have remained the same or even improved during menopause.

Pat is a forty-six-year-old mother of two young sons who says her sex life has always been great. During perimenopause, which started for her at age forty-five, she noticed a decrease in her level of lubrication. She discussed it with her nurse practitioner, and they decided that she needed a low-dosage natural estrogen pill, which took care of her problem. She has not experienced any changes in arousal or intensity of climaxes.

Betty, a fifty-one-year-old gay African-American woman, says she and her partner are having the best sex of their lives. They both entered menopause around the same time and actually seem to be experiencing the same symptoms. They are eating more soy and exercising daily to help them deal with hot flashes.

Some women confess that their greatest fear about menopause is related to wondering whether their partners would still find them attractive. Sally, forty-eight, has just started menopause. She says at first she was too embarrassed to discuss her changing sexual needs with her partner, who happens to be only thirty-seven years old. Although they have enjoyed a great sex life, she didn't want to discuss her menopause symptoms because she felt that would emphasize the difference in their ages. She said she wasn't sure he was ready to hear what she had to say. But because she began to avoid sex due to vaginal dryness, she was forced to tell him what was happening. He was receptive to her feelings and offered to do whatever he could to help. They decided she needed more foreplay and she also started using a vaginal lubricant.

What African-American women in menopause are saying about their sex lives:

It's still good. I can't say I have as much energy. I'm still waiting for that post-menopausal zest to kick in. But we get there and I have no complaints. Not dealing with a period or worrying about pregnancy makes a difference.

I've had orgasms at twenty, thirty, forty, and fifty, but the best sex of my life is at age sixty. I feel free and my confidence is high. Nothing worries me anymore. Sex at sixty rocks!

Sex at menopause is different but better. I am not controlled by it anymore and now I really, really know what I want.

We have to work at finding the time to be together. Now more than ever, we plan romantic evenings. We also make sure we spend more time talking to each other and just cuddling.

My body isn't what it used to be and neither is his. We don't let that stop us. We know so much more about how to make each other feel good.

Other women expressed concern about the following in relation to their sexuality and their fears about feeling less desirable:

♦ Fear of gaining weight
♦ Fear of looking old and unattractive
♦ Fear of developing skin problems
♦ Fear of sagging breasts
♦ Fear that their sexual partner might compare their body to the way it was when they were younger
♦ Fear that it would be harder to reach climax
♦ Fear of not feeling sexy

Discuss these issues with your caregiver and make a commitment to address each with an action plan. Become more active in toning your body, try harder to lose weight, adjust your skincare regime, improve your nutrition, and boost your self-esteem with affirmations. Think about what you can do to recapture that sexy feeling again. For us, sex starts in the mind. Share your feelings with a close friend or advisor who will help you resolve your feelings and support you in making the changes necessary to looking and feeling good. When you are ready once again, take the time to talk with your sexual partner about your feelings.

Dr. Barbara Levy's Perspective

Medically, disorders of sexual function are divided into four separate areas: 1) libido, or interest and fantasy about sexual behaviors; 2) arousal disorders, or the inability to lubricate and engorge despite an interest in sexual activity; 3) anorgasmia, the inability to achieve a climax; and 4) pain disorders—either pain with initial penetration or pain with deep intercourse. Each of these areas may be a problem for menopausal women. Sometimes it is difficult to figure out what the original problem was, as each of these areas can feed into the others, creating a snowball effect.

For example, if sex is painful, it will become increasingly difficult to be interested in an activity that hurts! None of us are such gluttons for punishment that we relish doing things that are uncomfortable. When sex hurts, we begin to avoid behaviors that will lead to sexual activity. Also, the fear of pain will change our physiological responses and create difficulty with arousal. The lack of lubrication of the vagina increases discomfort, so we become less and less interested. We may also avoid intimacy and cuddling for fear that our partners will become aroused and initiate sexual contact. Finally, without proper arousal and engorgement of the blood vessels supplying the vulva, vagina, and clitoris, orgasm is difficult to achieve. Women report feeling "dead down there." The nerve endings are not getting the message properly.

The physical changes that occur with estrogen deficiency may set up this cascade of events. However, diminishing sexual pleasure is not inevitable as we age and lose estrogen. This is definitely a situation where "you lose it if you don't use it." Consistent sexual activity and arousal will reduce the physical thinning of the skin in the vulva and vagina. Regular exercise also increases the blood flow to our genital tissues and increases sexual sensation. For those women who cannot use estrogen replacement or who choose not to, local estrogen in the form of a vaginal ring, creams, or extremely low-dose vaginal tablets will provide excellent relief of dryness without elevating circulating blood levels of estrogen.

In addition, many of us create much of the outside dryness by washing the genitals with soap. These tissues are extremely sensitive and designed to be quite oily. When we scrub them with a loofah, washcloth, or even our hands using harsh soaps, we deplete the oil from the skin and permit urine and sweat to penetrate into the tissues. These substances are irritating and set up a chronic inflammation, causing itching and significant discomfort. We may get away with scrubbing with antibacterial soaps when we are young. However, as we mature, our skin becomes dryer and more sensitive. You wouldn't think of treating a baby's bottom so harshly.

I recommend avoiding all soaps and harsh chemicals. Wash the vagina by splashing it with water. The oil in the skin will create a barrier to the germs and allow them to wash away fairly easily. If you have trouble with urine leaking, wear a pad all day. If you have continued irritation, you will be amazed at how much relief you will get by coating the vulva with Crisco or Bag Balm after you bathe or shower every day. I know it sounds crazy, but it really works wonders!

Smoking, diabetes, high blood pressure, and many of the medications used to treat these conditions may alter libido and sexual function in women as well as men. If you have noticed an abrupt change in your sexual feelings, discuss this situation with your physician. It may well be that a physical condition exists that is diminishing your responsiveness, or the medication you are taking may be the culprit.

Depression, the second most common disorder among women in the world, can be a serious threat to healthy sexual function. Diminished interest in sex is a hallmark symptom of depression. The medications to treat depression are notorious for their sexual side effects. The fluoxetine (Prozac) class of drugs, called serotonin reuptake inhibitors (Zoloft, Paxil, and Celexa also belong to this category) can affect both libido and orgasm. These problems seem to be most common when the drugs are first begun, and frequently diminish with time. Some people, though, do not recover their sexual feelings while on these medications. As a clinician, it is often difficult to determine whether the depression is inadequately treated, leading to continuing symptoms, or whether the drugs themselves are responsible for the lack of sexual interest and orgasmic ability.

Other forms of therapy for depression may be useful, rather than resorting to medication. There are some tricks to diminishing side effects if medication is essential to controlling depressive symptoms. Adding a second type of antidepressant, buproprion—the one used to help people quit smoking—may reverse some of the effects of the SSRIs and permit resumption of normal sexual function. Taking the herb gingko biloba daily may also be beneficial. Finally, the addition of a drug for anxiety called buspirinone (Buspar) may also help.

Sometimes the depression women experience is related to a history of physical or sexual violence in the past. More than 25 percent of women in this country have been victims of domestic violence or sexual abuse at some time in their lives. These experiences tend to fester within us and create significant problems with sexual arousal. We learn to dissociate what is happening to our bodies from our consciousness during these episodes in order to survive emotionally. That dissociation, however, may persist, making us unable to feel. Sexual activity may rekindle fear, anxiety, and even panic reactions (usually unrecognized), which diminish or even completely erase any positive emotions and feelings we have with our current partner. This makes it very difficult to feel sensual or aroused. If you have been a victim of sexual or physical violence at some time in your life and have difficulty with sex drive, arousal, orgasm, or pain, it will be important to find a health care provider with whom you feel safe. Your sex life will not improve until you can understand the reactions your body is having and learn to overcome the fear and loathing that sexual intimacy may evoke.

Most of us do not know that women have a physiological sexual response very similar to men. When we are aroused, our tissues become engorged, the vagina secretes a thin, clear fluid that lubricates the tissues, and the vagina increases in length by about 30 percent. Women who experience pain with deep penetration often tell me "it feels like he's hitting something." Generally, this is a result of vaginal penetration before the female partner is sufficiently aroused. Some of our partners are anxious for intercourse (especially if they took Viagra an hour ago!) and forget our need for foreplay to become aroused. Men are generally more easily aroused than we are. We need a safe, cozy atmosphere, romance, cuddling, and non-genital touching to get us in the mood. If we try to make him happy by accommodating him before we're ready, pain often results. If deep pain persists, it is important to check with a gynecologist for evaluation.

As we mature, couples need a bit more communication to be able to satisfy both partners without pain. Sometimes that means changing positions to avoid pressure on a painful joint, and sometimes it means wining, dining, and candlelight to help create the romance that helps us to feel sensual.

Sometimes we don't feel sensual because we are dissatisfied with our appearance or the appearance of our partner. It is hard for us to be sexy when we hate our bodies. If our partner has gained weight or smells bad, if our bodies have changed a great deal either from illness or just aging, we may not feel attractive even to ourselves. These problems require a lot of discussion and communication to resolve.

Inability to achieve orgasm is a difficult problem for many women. Culturally, some of us were raised to believe that our bodies are sinful and not for pleasure. When we have those words and judgments floating around in our minds, it is very hard to allow ourselves to feel sensual and turned on. Physical pleasure makes us feel guilty. Counseling and discussion with a trained professional therapist will probably be needed to help overcome these taboos of our upbringing. In order to learn how to experience orgasm, women must be comfortable exploring their bodies and learning for themselves what areas are sensitive and pleasurable. Our partners can help us in this. However, until we are comfortable feeling pleasure for ourselves, we won't be able to communicate well with a lover.

Tips for being sensuous

Learn to love yourself. That seems like a simple task, but it is not. Women are raised to care for everyone else before considering their own needs. Many of us don't even recognize our needs anymore. Sensuality requires time, relaxation, and a calm, centered spirit. We can achieve these things by setting boundaries at work and at home to create space and time for us. Exercise is essential to our physical health, stamina, and sense of well-being. If you have not been exercising, begin with walking and maybe some light handheld weights. You'll be amazed at how much better you can feel after just two or three weeks of gentle activity. If you are unable to walk, consider aqua aerobics, yoga, swimming, biking, or some other activity. The increased physical stamina will improve your sex life enormously! Find music, scents, colors, and fabrics that make you feel good.

Each of us has a slightly different temperament, so what works for me won't necessarily be right for you. Some women love luxuriating in a bubble bath (be sure to coat the genital tissues with Crisco to keep the chemicals off sensitive skin) or soaking in a hot tub. Whatever activity helps you feel beautiful and alive, do it. Your body will soon learn to recognize the signals—the candlelight, the music, the scent—whatever works for you. You will find that these activities begin to make you feel aroused and sensual. Whether or not you have a partner, sexual activity often follows.

Some women enjoy watching sexually arousing movies or tapes. Some women prefer romantic scenes. Watching videos is a powerful stimulant for many people. There is no reason why we shouldn't enjoy these if they help to stimulate healthy sexual activity.

Did you know…

Did you know 25 percent of women in early menopausal years report problems with vaginal dryness?

Did you know that once problems with vaginal dryness and hot flashes are resolved, 75 percent of menopausal women report that their sexual functioning is fine?

Did you know only 32 percent of menopausal women complain of painful intercourse?

Did you know 70 percent of women report no decrease in sexual desire during menopause?

TESTOSTERONE AND SEXUAL FUNCTIONING

The impact of deficient testosterone levels on our libido is something else to consider. New information shows that many women may need testosterone supplementation to correct sexual problems. The Black women I come in contact with don't have a clue about the role that testosterone plays in our sexual functioning, and conflicting reports contribute to their confusion. Dr. Susan Rako believes testosterone is as important for healthy sexual functioning for women as it is for men. She states, "A woman's normal physiology includes the production of a critical amount of testosterone, essential to her normal sexual development, to the healthy functioning of virtually all tissues in her body, and to her experience of vital energy and sexual libido."

It has only been in the last five years that the popular press has started printing articles about women's sexuality at midlife. Because of increased media coverage, many women are becoming more aware that solutions are available. We haven't caught up with the level of attention focused on impotence and Viagra, but we are getting there. Remember, it's quite possible you may not require any assistance in this area, but if you do, talk to your doctor about any sexual difficulties and gather the appropriate information.

There are some possible side effects of testosterone:

♦ Increase in appetite
♦ Weight gain
♦ Facial hair
♦ Acne
♦ Hair loss
♦ Deepening of the voice

Adjusting the dose can usually eliminate these problems.

My primary problem in the sexual area has been vaginal dryness. I asked about vaginal creams, but Dr. Levy suggested Estring. It is a small plastic ring that is easy to insert and lasts for ninety days. It releases a small amount of estrogen on a daily basis. Estring made a big difference and is not at all messy like creams or suppositories. I had to write down the date of insertion because it was so comfortable that I forgot about it. Eventually I switched to Vagifem, a tiny estrogen tablet that is inserted twice weekly. It is made by the same company, Pharmacia-Upjohn/Pfizer, and I like it much better than the ring. It's very easy to use and comes in a disposable applicator. Vagifem releases minute amounts of estrogen gradually, and I find that my level of lubrication is more consistent.

Some women report having hot flashes when they climax. Others state that their level of sexual satisfaction is improved. As with all aspects of menopause, the reactions are unique to each individual.

Unfortunately, little research has been done on sexual functioning during menopause. Many women report problems with vaginal dryness, but most say their overall sexual desire hasn't changed.

MENOPAUSE STRATEGIES

Sometimes it can be difficult to talk with your partner about sexual issues. I encourage you to schedule a weekly meeting to discuss your feelings. Each person must be prepared to really listen for at least ten minutes to the other person. Once you begin responding, you have to talk only about your feelings. This helps you own your feelings as well as making sure you do not become judgmental of your partner's concerns.

You might just want to vent. There are times when I just wanted to tell Lester that I had lost my bearings and how difficult it was for me to feel this way.

You might feel a need to stroked and touched just to reassure you that he cares about what you're going through. This is a time to say, "I just want you to hold me." If you just want some sympathy and support regarding your menopause or perimenopause issues, you should make that clear.

You might be ready to take a hard look at the problems and talk about what needs to be done. It has been my experience that men often want to do this step first. If what you need is a chance to focus on problems and come up with strategies to solve them, then you will need to take an entirely different approach.

Examples of what to say

I'm really struggling with this whole menopause thing. Over the past few weeks, I have had trouble sleeping and, as you may have noticed, it's hard for me to control my moods. I just want you to know that I'm working on this and it will get better. I want you to hang in here with me. Can you do that? Can you hold me right now? How do you feel about what I'm saying?

We need to talk about several things related to our sex life. I am experiencing some discomfort because of a lack of estrogen in my body right now. I will need more time to get aroused and will need additional lubrication. My doctor has suggested several other things that we can do to help me relax. Would you like to try some of them?

I had several discussions with my husband about my symptoms. I explained why I was having problems with vaginal dryness. He was surprised to learn that a lack of estrogen was responsible for so many of the problems that I was experiencing. As I discussed each problem with Dr. Levy, I would also discuss my treatment options with Lester so he could support me and work with me. Often, it was a trial-and-error process because each of us reacts differently to hormones and medications. We couldn't always predict how I was going to respond to new products and dosages.

I tell women to talk with their partners and explore their feelings or concerns about menopause. There are so many myths about this passage that each person has probably heard conflicting information over the years. If your partner's conditioning about menopause is negative, these things need to be brought out in the open. Many men seem concerned about how menopause will affect our sexual responses. They worry we are going to be different in some way. They don't know what to expect. It is helpful to allow them to express their feelings. It's also good to give them as much clear information as you can.

Dr. Levy asked me to appear with her on a local television news program, on a segment called "The Truth about Menopause." When the camera team came out, they filmed both Lester and me. He made several positive comments, but unfortunately they included the one negative comment he made on the show. But perhaps that made it easier for other men to express their fears to him. Once the program aired, several men approached Lester to discuss how they could help their wives. He has a much greater understanding of menopause than most men because of our discussions. He encourages other men to be patient and to improve their listening skills. I have to say that he has learned a lot and worked hard to understand what I was experiencing.

Many women report that sex after menopause is better. They attribute this to the fact that they are more comfortable with themselves, they feel confident with their own sexuality, and they have less pressure to deal with at home. Other women feel free because they don't have to worry about birth control, and others are relieved that they no longer have periods and any of the discomforts related to menstruation.

MY MENOPAUSAL STRATEGIES FOR ENHANCING SEXUAL ENJOYMENT
+ Taking more time for foreplay
+ Taking a steam bath together to get in the mood
+ Watching erotic movies together
+ Stimulating myself when necessary to keep the tissues healthy
+ Reading erotic books
+ Using sexual fantasies
+ Asking my husband to give me massages
+ Setting the mood with candles and romantic love songs
+ Going out dancing

Ask Dr. Levy

Q: Vaginal dryness can make it painful to have sex. How big a problem is vaginal dryness for women in menopause? Is it very common? What are the causes?

A: A decrease in estrogen causes a decrease in skin elasticity as well as decrease in secretions. Eliminate douching as well as soap.

Q: How does a lack of estrogen affect the sex drive?

A: Decreased blood flow to the vulva and vagina can decrease sensation as well as increase discomfort. Who wants to do something that doesn't feel good or even hurts? The more sexual activity women maintain, the less this is a problem.

Q: When is taking testosterone necessary?

A: There's no question that when women surgically lose their ovaries, they lose about 80 percent of their testosterone. The adrenal glands that sit above the kidneys make a little testosterone, but most of it comes from the ovaries. So surgically menopausal women have an abrupt dropoff in testosterone levels, and that can affect their libido and sense of well-being. It doesn't happen to everybody, and I don't know why. It may be because the adrenals actually produce more estrogen in some women. It may be because so much of our sexual function is cognitive. Good sex is about how we think about sex and how we feel about sex, and not so much about how our hormones stimulate us. In any case, testosterone replacement is definitely in order for women who have their ovaries removed, who have symptoms of just not feeling quite as well or as energetic. Testosterone levels begin to drop in our mid-forties, maybe even a little earlier than that, and some women seem to be very sensitive to that decrease. These testosterone levels do not diminish as estrogen is reduced at menopause. It's a much more subtle process. I think when in doubt and when a woman has a lot of symptoms and she comes in and says to me, "You know, I used to be this highly sexual person and it's really changed a lot," that's something I should examine.

If I check her estrogen levels and they are still normal, I do not have a problem with trying physiological levels of testosterone replacement. It can't be purchased in a drugstore. There is no prescription commercially available that is natural testosterone. The only way to get this hormone is by going to a compounding pharmacy, where the formulation is completed on the spot and tailored specifically for each individual. One percent or 2 percent testosterone in either an ointment or a cream gets absorbed in the inner wrist or inner thigh. The cream would sting a little bit if you put in on the vulva. The ointment can be placed directly on the vulva, and that's more direct stimulation for some people. Women who are having some sexual problems, even if they still possess their ovaries, should try to use this ointment. I don't necessarily just measure levels because I don't think that the labs are all that good at giving us answers.

Q: How do you know when you have enough testosterone?
A: A pea size every day for about two weeks ought to be plenty. If there's no change in how someone feels at that point, then I would say their feelings and their symptoms are not related to lack of testosterone. We should start looking at other things we can do to improve their symptoms.

Q: Are testosterone creams always effective for treating low sex drive?
A: They only work if low testosterone is the cause of low libido. It will not affect sex drive if the root cause is a poor relationship or poor communication with your partner.

Q: How does menopause affect the sex drive of most of your patients?

A: Age rather than hormonal status seems to be the bigger factor. People whose lives are well-balanced don't experience any problems.

Q: Is it true that women in menopause can expect body hair to decrease?

A: Overall, hair thins. Women in menopause can expect body hair to decrease everywhere. Body fat and hair distribution change as we age.

Q: Tell us about urinary incontinence. What causes it and is incontinence a big problem during menopause? Are Kegel exercises a good remedy for minor incontinence?

A: Yes. Kegel exercises are pelvic muscle exercises, and when done properly they teach a woman how to prevent urine loss when coughing, sneezing, or laughing by strengthening pubococcygeal muscles. These are the same muscles you use to release or stop urination. Practice involves tightening the muscles for ten seconds and relaxing them for twenty seconds several times a day. Then you alternate by tightening for twenty seconds and relaxing for ten. Increase practice gradually until you are doing about one hundred fifty repetitions per day.

Q: Are estrogen creams helpful for vaginal dryness?

A: Creams help vulvular and vaginal dryness. It is hard to absorb a consistent amount to obtain the other benefits of estrogen replacement therapy. All estrogens—patches, pills, creams, shots, ring, and implants—will improve vaginal dryness.

Q: Are yeast infections and bladder infections more common during menopause?

A: Yeast infections are not more common in menopause. Bladder infections increase without estrogen because the tissue surrounding the uterus as well as the bladder itself is thinner and more susceptible to injury. Yogurt containing live cultures can help to balance the bacteria and yeast throughout the body. Do not douche or wash with soap.

MENOPAUSE CALL TO ACTION

♦ Don't accept less than you deserve in your sex life during menopause.
♦ Take action at the first sign of a problem with your sexual response.
♦ Celebrate your sexuality.
♦ Be sensual and loving in your sexual encounters.
♦ Eliminate any fear about not being able to perform and enjoy sex.
♦ Recognize and tend to your sexual needs even when you don't have a partner.

CHAPTER 8

Complementary Medicine for Enhancing Wellness

AFRICAN-AMERICAN HEALING TRADITIONS

African-Americans have a long history tied to natural medicine and wellness. Centuries ago we were in the habit of relying on medicine women, healers, shamans, herbalists, and root doctors. During times in our past when we couldn't afford medical treatment, we sought home remedies and preventative health measures. Using natural remedies during midlife will take us back to our roots. All of us can probably remember a relative or extended family member who provided health-care remedies for the family. In the past, these remedies were sometimes seen as "old wives' tales," but now many people in this country are beginning to recognize the wisdom of natural or complementary medicine.

Some people call it alternative medicine, but Dr. Levy and I believe complementary medicine is the proper term because it reflects the true relationship between traditional and nontraditional medicine. These two types of medicine complement each other. There are times when one is better than the other based on our health-care needs. At other times, we need to use both to help our bodies heal. This chapter will explore how you can use complementary remedies, exercise, and nutrition to manage your perimenopause/menopause symptoms and enhance your midlife transition by achieving optimal health and wellness.

As we explore methods of natural and complementary medicine, we should be aware that the definition of a drug is any substance ingested into the body for the purpose of treating or preventing illness or other conditions. Just because a product is advertised as natural or because we can buy it over the counter does not mean it should not be handled with care. Natural and plant substances have the potential to be either helpful or harmful because they have agents in them with the power to impact our bodies. We should consult with a health care professional, a certified herbalist, nutritionist, naturopath, or holistic doctor before trying to medicate ourselves.

Capturing and utilizing some of the old "down home" ways of healing that are recognized as effective medicine today is a good strategy for us. Can you think of any home remedies or natural healing strategies used by your family? I have many memories of my mom using natural healing. I grew up in Detroit, where it gets very cold. My mother made us take cod liver oil every morning during the winter when the temperature was below zero for weeks. My grandmother made her family take castor oil for the same purpose. Eating oatmeal for breakfast every day was a must because she believed it was the healthiest food in the world. We had at least three servings of vegetables each day and lots of fiber-rich foods like rice, beans, and corn. She canned fruits and vegetables in the fall, and she believed in using fresh garlic and herbs for cooking. She did not use much salt. We didn't eat a lot of meat, mainly because we couldn't afford it, and butter was considered a luxury.

It was only as we got older, our family income increased, and our lifestyle changed that we began to eat the typical American diet of fast food and lots of meat. Complex carbohydrates were served with every meal and we were given specific foods when we were sick, such as peaches, ginger ale, chicken broth, and homemade soup.

Assessing Your Level of Health

How do you define good health? This is an important question to answer before you can assess where you are in terms of your perceived level of health.

+ How healthy do you think you are?
+ How healthy do you want to be at midlife?
+ What do you do on a daily basis to maintain good health?
+ Are you motivated to work on your health at midlife?

Wellness Factors

Wellness is based on many factors as follows:

+ Eating habits
+ Weight management
+ Level of body fat
+ Flexibility
+ Strength
+ Use of vitamins/minerals
+ Use of herbal supplements
+ Frequency of exercise
+ Stress load
+ Relaxation methods
+ Frequency of smoking and drinking alcohol
+ Spiritual philosophy
+ Positive relationships
+ Ability to manage time
+ Meaningful work and/or creative outlets

Take some time to evaluate yourself on each factor listed above and then commit to making changes to increase your level of wellness. Educate yourself and then change your habits. Do you have positive relationships and a supportive network? Women who have close friends cope better with challenges.

According to the American Academy of Anti-Aging, the characteristics we associate with aging can really be attributed to lifestyle habits. What habits do you have that might be causing you to age prematurely?

Cultural Values

Our culture assigns meanings to events and circumstances and the way we interpret them. The meaning attached to wellness is culturally determined, and there are differences within our culture from group to group. The way I describe being physically fit will be quite different for you. But no matter where we stand on the true meaning of wellness, all of us want to be healthy and happy. In order to achieve and maintain our health at the highest level, we need to develop lifestyle habits that help us nourish our bodies and prevent illness.

African-American women do not make preventive practices a focus in our lives. Simply eating differently, exercising, and handling stress are keys to better health and longevity for us. These are the lifestyle factors that cause us to die of heart disease, diabetes, and stroke. We must face the fact that our major health problems are often preventable and our poor choices cause us to get sick. Getting older is inevitable, but aging can be slowed down by adequate exercise, good nutrition, and learning how to relax.

Health care professionals tell us we are victims of the "quicker and sicker" syndrome. Disease conditions manifest quickly and make us sicker than they make white women. It doesn't help that we tend to wait until we are faced with a medical challenge before working on our health. In this chapter, as we explore the benefits of proper nutrition, exercise, stress management, and complementary medicine, we will show you how to improve your health at midlife. We review and discuss some of the well-known schools of thought, providing you with an overview so that you can make a decision about how to incorporate some of these strategies in your life. The information shared will help you evaluate your wellness and then put together your own Personal Health Success Plan.

Medical anthropology suggests that our bodies adapted to food deprivation over the centuries by holding on to every single nutrient to survive. Because we come from a group of people who lived in Africa, a very hot climate, and then were enslaved in the South, our bodies have evolved to a point where we have a tendency to retain salt. We were forced to eat poor quality pork and smoked foods, the scraps and leftovers given to us during slavery times to keep from starving. Over time we developed a craving for foods that we know are unhealthy. Some folks call "chitlins" a delicacy, but I have a friend who says every time we eat them we put one foot closer to the grave. If these theories about how we developed poor eating habits and developed a cultural predisposition to be unhealthy are true, then we must adjust our lifestyle habits accordingly. Think about it. It's possible that we as a people are predisposed to be overweight and hypertensive. That makes proper nutrition and exercise more critical.

Doc Talk — An Interview with Dr. Beverly Yates

I contacted Dr. Beverly Yates, a naturopathic physician who lives in San Rafael, California. I sought her advice for African-American women in midlife after reading her book, *Heart Health for Black Women*. She explained how negative emotions and memories of great pain and suffering may be passed down through generations. Her discussion of how slavery impacted our well-being today was thought provoking. She believes Black women have heart problems arising from psychological and emotional issues as well as lifestyle habits. These feelings are tied to the aftereffects of major suffering that have been carried over from our maternal ancestors, women who coped with their children and spouses being sold and their families destroyed. They lived with unimaginable daily heartbreak. This tremendous sorrow still impacts our psyche today. It is a legacy, but we can break the cycle after increasing our awareness of why we behave the way we do.

Because of living with what she calls "sustained stress," without outlets for expressing our feelings, we are in the habit of holding everything in while we let others tell us how strong we are. She openly discusses some of her own feelings of rage and how she learned to cope. We are predisposed to develop heart disease unless we make new choices about our health. In her practice, she teaches women how to take a natural approach to midlife transition. She cautions "against a knee-jerk reaction to taking estrogen during midlife without exploring all our options." She also talks about how our history in this country, including our recent past, influences our health. She says, "Black women need to give themselves the gift of liberation."

Her remarks led me to reflect on my childhood influences and how what I learned affects my "health image" today. I was taught some good habits about being healthy and active. My mom has always believed it is important to maintain an active life. At seventy-three years of age, she bowls four to five nights a week and has scores that are almost on par with professional bowlers. Before she retired from working at Children's Hospital of Michigan, she was ranked as the best hitter on her department's baseball team well into her fifties and early sixties.

As a child and adolescent, I was a tomboy and she always supported my athletic activities. I was encouraged to play basketball, play volleyball, and go jogging. Every summer, I enjoyed rowboating, racing, and canoeing at camp. I started out my young adult years living an active lifestyle, used to go dancing several nights a week, and jogged five days a week for fun. In my thirties I would ride my bike about twenty miles per week. As I reached the age of forty, I allowed other obligations to take priority. I forgot the lessons I had been taught about the benefits of being active. This might be true for you as well. At midlife, a time when it is most crucial for us to move our bodies, we may have ten to twelve years of leading a sedentary lifestyle. Many women tell me they don't have much time for themselves, and when they do, they are usually too exhausted to work out. We forget that exercising will not only help us have more energy, it will also help our bodies adjust to the changes of menopause/perimenopause. I want to help you pinpoint the time in your life when you began to see exercise as a chore instead of a way to enjoy life.

Our cultural conditioning also included using spiritual techniques like fasting to improve health. We were taught that God wants us to be healthy in mind, body, and spirit, and gluttony is a deadly sin. Many of us were raised to believe in the power of fasting to rid our bodies of toxins and to help us become more spiritually aware at certain times of the year. At my church, our minister encouraged families to fast together. But there are other cultural barriers to wellness.

Barriers to wellness in our communities
♦ Lack of knowledge about good nutrition
♦ Cultural tolerance for obesity and a lack of knowledge about the health benefits of weight loss
♦ Cultural values placed on eating high-fat foods
♦ Community education programs promoting wellness are not culturally appropriate
♦ An abundance of food was seen as a sign of prosperity
♦ At major celebrations and small family/community gatherings, feasting on favorite foods was expected. It was impolite to turn down food even if you were not hungry

♦ Family hiking vacations or other active leisure-time activities are not common

HOLISTIC MEDICINE

Holistic medicine is based on the premise that the body is capable of healing itself and that treating the whole person includes the body, mind, and spirit. Patients and caregivers work together to help discover the cause of diseases. As patients, we have to be accountable for our own health, and we must choose to improve our health by changing our lifestyle.

What will you do to learn more about holistic medicine? Do you know where to locate a holistic health practitioner in your area?

Exercising regularly is one of the most important and beneficial things we can do to improve our health and to maintain wellness. Exercise is a remedy as well as a method of prevention. In order to have a healthy heart, you must take part in an aerobic activity a minimum of three times per week for at least thirty minutes. Strength training with weights is also highly recommended for women over forty to build more muscle mass, strength, and healthy bones, and to manage weight.

> **"The Ancient Egyptians did not separate the mind and body. Instead they would describe organs of the body as having mental or spiritual qualities, though they also understood that there was a unity between the body, mind, emotions and spirit."**
> —**Marcellus A. Walker, M.D. and Kenneth B. Singleton, M.D.,** *Natural Health for African-American,*

Select an activity and commit to at least four hours per week

	How long?	What day?
___Walking	_____	_____
___Golfing	_____	_____
___Yoga	_____	_____
___Bike riding	_____	_____
___Weight lifting	_____	_____
___Jogging	_____	_____
___Tennis	_____	_____
___Handball	_____	_____
___Swimming	_____	_____

For those of us who are in menopause, exercise is as important to us as drinking water. In my early forties, I decided to start lifting weights again. This time I decided to hire a personal trainer and worked out three times a week. It was the best investment of my life, and Juli and I became the best of friends. I learned how to breathe properly and developed excellent form.

I enjoyed weight lifting for several reasons. I liked building my upper body strength and I loved the muscle definition that I was getting in my legs, thighs, and arms. I also became hooked on the good feelings that came to me when I pushed myself.

My current exercise routine includes walking two miles three days a week on my treadmill and using free weights to work on my chest, back, biceps, and triceps. I also have an aerobic rider, which is great for toning the upper body. I try to get on it three times per week for twenty minutes. Now I practice yoga for thirty minutes four times a week in the morning. I am in love with it, and I highly recommend it.

My morning exercise routine isn't consistent because often don't I get up early enough to do it before starting my day. When the weather is nice, I prefer to walk outside at Seward Park, which is seven minutes away from my house. Here in Seattle we treasure the few months of sunshine given to us and we try to spend as much time as possible outdoors. Although I prefer a morning workout to set the tone for my day, working out after work is easier for me to fit into my schedule, so I often do so in the evenings. Maintaining a routine when I am out of town is also another challenge. We all have our specific challenges to focus on during this journey to becoming healthy and fit.

It's helpful to keep fit by doing a variety of activities that you really enjoy. I like to dance, canoe, bike ride, and play basketball. Most of us will spend more time on activities we find enjoyable. A lifelong goal has been to join a women's rowing team. One day I know I will make the commitment to do it. I have been considering taking golf lessons so that my husband and I can play together. He loves golfing, sailing, handball, and tennis, but I'm not proficient in any of those activities. We want to have an activity that we can enjoy together.

At this time of my life, regular exercise has become even more crucial to my mental health. It gives me energy and enthusiasm but also helps keep my moods stabilized. I have a tendency to slow down after missing several days, or find myself easily irritated. I am still struggling with the level of commitment necessary to make exercise a daily habit so that I will do it automatically without any inner debate.

After sixty to ninety days, most people can significantly improve their ability to cope with stress by working on their mind, body, and spirit. I counsel my clients to make lifestyle changes in diet, exercise, relaxation, and leisure activities. Incremental changes are easy, and small successes can motivate us to set larger goals.

Benefits of exercise

♦ Helps maintain proper weight
♦ Helps ensure a healthy heart
♦ Builds strength and endurance
♦ Facilitates a good mood
♦ Increases energy level
♦ Builds muscle
♦ Keeps us feeling young and vibrant
♦ Helps to lower blood sugar levels and improves the way our bodies use insulin, so exercise helps manage diabetes
♦ Enhances circulation
♦ Lowers cholesterol

STRENGTH TRAINING IS KEY

It has been proven that muscle burns fat faster. You must lift weights in order to lose weight. Six months of weight training can make a drastic change in your health.

Miriam Nelson, Ph.D., is the author of *Strong Women Stay Young* and teaches at the school of Nutrition of Science and Policy at Tufts University. Dr. Nelson designed a program of strength training where women worked out twice a week at home for a year. Many of these women were over the age of sixty and they still made dramatic improvements in their health. It is apparently never too late. Girlfriends, let's get started. It is time to do ourselves a big favor and get fit.

Did you know...

Did you know muscle burns up to fifty more calories per hour than fat does?
Did you know adding three pounds of muscle would help you burn an extra 120 calories per day?

Did you know a study at Harvard University showed that people lived two years longer if they engaged in moderate exercise?

Did you know people who are physically active tend to be less anxious and exhibit more self-confidence?

Did you know after age thirty, we tend to lose 3 percent to 6 percent of our muscle mass per decade?

Did you know exercise improves your body's ability to process insulin?

Did you know when your system uses insulin effectively, it processes carbohydrates more efficiently, which stabilizes blood sugar and reduces hunger between meals?

Did you know some fat in your diet is necessary because fat insulates our bodies, provides a cushion for our organs, and stores energy?

BODY IMAGE AND EXERCISE

The skin on our breasts usually begins to sag during menopause. This change is caused by a loss of elasticity of the muscles and ligaments that support breast tissue. Doing exercises that tone the muscles of your chest and upper back can alleviate this problem. If you're concerned about your appearance as you get older, then daily exercise is the key. It's the only way to maintain a well-toned and fit body.

SELF-TALK AND EXERCISE

One of the biggest problems we face is the way we talk to ourselves when we don't succeed with our exercise programs. It's important to avoid putting yourself down and falling into the trap of self-hatred when that happens. Our performance falls even lower when we beat ourselves up mentally. Changing self-talk about being active is the first step. Our first tendency is to immediately change our performance or behavior. But we must talk to ourselves in a different way. Our minds are so powerful that our behavior will automatically change once we control our self-talk. This is why affirmations are so powerful in helping us address all of our perimenopausal/menopausal needs.

Conduct a week-long exercise to help you become more aware of the quality of your thoughts. Every time you say or think something negative about your body, write it down on an index card. At the end of the week, write down positive self-talk statements to substitute for the negative thoughts. Boost yourself and visualize the new behaviors you want to adopt.

Tell yourself that you enjoy exercising on the treadmill three times per week for thirty minutes or more. Say it over and over. Record each session in a notebook or journal. When you skip sessions, don't put yourself down in any way. Just tell yourself what you intend to do next week. The technique of looking forward helps you control negative self-talk, focuses on positive end results, and builds a positive expectancy for your future. It sounds simple, but many methods of mind control and self-discipline are based on simple principles. When you change the way you think, you will change the way you act.

> **"The active life is not one of denial and deprivation, nor is it one of pain and hurt. It is a joyful experience, an affirmation of what we can be physically, mentally, socially, and spiritually."**
>
> *—American College of Sports Medicine*

Develop an exercise action plan by first listing the barriers to developing an active lifestyle.

♦ What keeps you from working out?

♦ What are the solutions to your barriers?

Design affirmations for each solution.

If lack of time is a barrier, write an affirmation to take the time to work out. If you need support, write an affirmation about getting a workout partner. If you aren't sure about what you want to achieve with your plan, write an affirmation about exploring different activities and routines until you find one that suits you.

Use the following affirmations to help affirm the benefits of working out on a regular basis.

AFFIRMATIONS

- I am healthy, strong, and physically fit.
- I always make exercising a priority in my life.
- Exercising daily adds great joy to my life. It's fun and I get tremendous satisfaction from moving my body.
- It thrills me to be fit and firm. I look good and feel good.
- I have a positive expectancy of working out three times every week and I believe every setback is temporary.
- I am hooked on the wonderful feelings I get from exercising.

AEROBICS 101

Aerobic activities keep your heart healthy and include activities such as jogging, swimming, cross-country skiing, hiking, rowing, stair climbing, and dancing.

The American College of Sports Medicine suggests a minimum of three aerobic workouts of twenty minutes or more three times per week. Other experts say two sessions per week is the minimum. All sources agree that maintaining a consistent routine is most important.

SELECTING A GOOD EXERCISE VIDEO

♦ Instructions should be clear.

♦ Safety measures should be discussed so that you understand how to avoid hurting yourself.

♦ Check the exercise video at your local video store or library first to make sure you will enjoy it before buying it.

♦ Make sure the tape has been certified by one of the following by organizations:

  • Aerobics & Fitness Association of America
  • American College of Sports Medicine
  • The American Council on Exercise

A good exercise program is a combination of aerobic exercise, strength training, and flexibility-enhancing activities such as yoga or stretching.

Life Lesson

What did you do for exercise as a young girl? Remember how we used to jump rope, play hopscotch, and do the hula hoop? We were active and we had lots of fun. We need to remember the joy of playing. Exercise can be fun again. Exercise is also a mind game. Start playing the game by thinking about and visualizing the fantastic results you will get. Feel your body getting stronger and leaner.

YOGA

Yoga provides many benefits. It helps to tone and strengthen our bodies while improving our endurance and flexibility. There are other benefits as well, such as aligning the way energy moves through our body. You start practicing yoga slowly and build as you become stronger and more flexible.

Yoga helps relieve stress and helps prevent disease. It helps increase muscle tone and spiritual awareness.

Yoga practice takes you through a series of body movements called asanas. There are many types of yoga. One of the most popular types in this country is called hatha yoga. I have been amazed at how much of a workout yoga provides. I take a class several mornings a week called *Inhale* with Steve Ross on Oprah's Oxygen channel. I started slowly and increased my level of participation each week. At the writing of this book, I am up to forty-five minutes. Try it! Besides helping you tone your body and enhance your concentration and balance, yoga just makes you feel good. African-American women all over this country are discovering the joys of yoga.

♦ Yoga builds focus, strength, and coordination.
♦ Yoga improves posture.
♦ Yoga releases tension.
♦ Yoga helps you lose weight.
♦ Yoga builds stamina.
♦ Yoga helps you align mind, body, and spirit.

Exercise Readiness Exam: What Is Your Score?

Keep score as follows:

Give yourself one point for each time you exercise over a period of ninety days. Deduct a point for each time you miss a session. The maximum number of points to be deducted in a week is three.

Exercise Readiness Exam point scale

36 points or more is	perfect
32 through 35	outstanding
27 through 31	excellent
20 through 26	good
15 through 19	fair
14 or less	needs improvement

Self-evaluation

+ What are your goals for exercising?
+ Do you have health problems that might interfere with your fitness regimen?
+ Are you willing to commit to a weekly program that fits your lifestyle?
+ Will you invest in the proper shoes and props to help you exercise?
+ Have you decided on the type of physical activity that you want to do?

Increase your Exercise Readiness Exam score by achieving a goal of exercising three times every week. Keep it up until your score improves.

CHAPTER 9

Success Strategies for a Healthier Life

BLACK WOMEN AND THE WEIGHT ISSUE

I don't need to go into the mechanics of counting calories and figuring out our level of body fat. We know all of this information, but many of us are not applying the knowledge. I'm overweight, and you know if you are as well. At midlife, it is time for us to resolve this problem once and for all. As of this writing, I have joined Weight Watchers along with my entire menopause group. We are committing to learning good eating habits and focusing on long-term goals. Get with your menopause support group and help support one another to conquer your issues with weight.

African-American women are disproportionally overweight, especially after age forty. We have to deal with how obesity, a risk factor for each of our high-risk medical conditions, negatively impacts our health. If weight is an issue for you as it is for me, let's look at what we can do to overcome this challenge. Recognizing that food provides pleasure, understanding we may be using food to satisfy emotional needs, being aware of the role that muscle plays in burning fat, and putting the focus on food management and long-term health and fitness are all principles to help us deal effectively with the weight issue. Let's proclaim perimenopause and menopause as our time to "take care of business."

There are several requirements for a successful weight-loss program:

♦ Eat lots of fiber.

♦ Fill up on complex carbohydrates.

♦ Increase your consumption of low-fat foods and learn how to cook traditional soul food with less fat and sugar.

♦ Eat several servings of fresh fruit and vegetables every day.

♦ Exercise with a combination of activities for aerobic exercise and weight training. Burn fat and build muscle.

♦ Get emotional support from a family member or friend.

♦ Develop a philosophy about eating based on principles that make sense to you. It might be a combination of several schools of thought or programs that you customize for yourself.

♦ Monitor your progress. Make a chart. Track your progress in a journal or on a map or poster. Display it prominently as a reminder.

♦ Don't let momentary setbacks frustrate you. Get back with the plan as soon as possible.

♦ Build a more active lifestyle.

♦ Increase your knowledge about what makes your body burn fat faster.

♦ When you get discouraged, remember just a loss of 5 to 10 percent of your total body weight decreases the risk of heart disease and diabetes and lowers your blood pressure.

♦ Keep a food diary. Write down everything you eat.

♦ Set smaller incremental goals to lose ten or fifteen pounds. Once you reach your interim goal, reset it.

♦ Eat more seafood.

♦ Plan to eat several vegetarian meals each week.

♦ Drink at least eighty ounces of water daily.

CHINESE MEDICINE AND WEIGHT LOSS

According to Henry C. Lu, author of *Chinese Natural Cures*, obesity is caused by several factors, including imbalance between organs. As we eat food to satisfy our taste buds and ignore what our bodies need to be healthy, we select foods that throw the body out of balance. He suggests the following tips on losing weight:

- Eat soups with small amounts of meat and lots of vegetables. He recommends beef soup, mung bean soup, mushroom soup, and chicken soup.
- Cut the fat from your meats before cooking them and boil the meat for twenty to thirty minutes. Rinse the meat with cold water before warming it.
- Drink green tea daily. It helps to reduce the impact of fat in the body.
- Get rid of water in the body by cooling the body with certain foods such as bitter gourd, which can be put in soup or tea. Fresh ginger and mung beans also help the body to eliminate water.
- Assist your kidneys in functioning properly by eating liver, mussels, animal kidneys, and shrimp. These foods act as a tonic for the kidneys.
- Eat foods that keep the body in balance, promote urination and elimination, and nourish the internal organs. These simple principles assist the body in returning to balance and facilitate long-term weight loss.

MANAGING STRESS AND LOSING WEIGHT

Coping with the stressors in our lives will also help us lose weight. If you have a tendency to be an emotional eater, take care of those stressors and it will be easier to lose weight.

In the early 1980s, while in graduate school, I decided the holistic approach to wellness was the best avenue for success, and I counseled women individually and in groups on how to manage the stress in their lives. We know stress takes a toll on every system in the body. In order to withstand the stress caused by the complexity of our lives, our bodies need to pull on reserves constantly. A proper diet, exercise, and relaxation replenish these reserves.

Life Lesson

Every Black woman has insightful stories about how she handles stress. Many of us are experts at coping with the stressors in our lives and moving on. Some of us are stress seekers and we thrive on stress in a positive manner. At other times, the stressors in our lives build up to a point where we lose control and our behavior leads to some chaotic times.

To stay on top of stress during menopause, we need to increase our awareness of what causes stress and how the impact may be intensified by the changes inherent to menopause. Stress is caused not only by our response to situations outside our control but also by self-imposed pressure. We know what troubles us and how we respond to unanticipated stress. Educating ourselves and preparing our minds and bodies for menopause will help eliminate some of the stressors tied to the Second Half of Life. See yourself as a "stress buster" who adapts to any unexpected stress and responds to daily stressors with a positive attitude and a winning approach. Relax and renew your reserves. Set priorities and follow your plan. Taking sixty-second stress breaks and visualizing peaceful scenes can often give you the mental break you need to conquer the next challenge with gusto!

HERBS

There are herbal remedies to help us deal with stress and menopausal symptoms. Using the right combination of herbs to help the body fight and prevent illness is a strategy that has been around for centuries. Herbs improve body chemistry, boost the immune system, eliminate toxins, and enhance internal balance. The use of herbs as complementary medicine has become more popular as research studies document their power to assist the body in healing.

Most herbs will not be powerful enough as a tea and should be taken as a liquid extract or capsule. Some herbs help us handle stress more efficiently by relaxing us and helping to calm the nervous system during menopause. These include chamomile, valerian root, lavender, and hops. Please note that lavender causes headaches in some women.

> **African slaves smuggled herbs in their clothing and hair to the countries where they were taken.**

HERBS FOR MENOPAUSE SYMPTOMS

Black Cohosh has been found to be effective in reducing or even eliminating hot flashes. It also helps to relax our muscles and blood vessels. It contains phytoestrogens.

Hawthorne Berry, a heart tonic, helps to lower blood pressure. It is a good remedy for night sweats and flashing. It also helps to strengthen the arteries.

Shepherd's Purse helps to lower heat in the body while serving as a relaxant.

Sage acts as an antioxidant, and because it reduces sweating, it helps curb hot flashes. It is also beneficial as a brain tonic, since it enhances memory.

Alfalfa helps to balance hormones and lower cholesterol, and operates in a way that is similar to soy.

Asian Ginseng is known as an anti-stress herb. Often hot flashes are aggravated by stress, so it stands to reason that Asian ginseng would be helpful. It has also been found to have a positive impact on vaginal dryness.

The following are herbs, vitamins, and minerals believed to be helpful for our special health risks of obesity, heart disease, and diabetes. This information is for educational purposes only and you should consult with a certified herbalist or naturopathic physician before using herbs to cope with your menopausal symptoms and conditions.

Obesity

+ **Vitamin B-6** operates as a diuretic during weight loss.
+ **Lecithin** granules help move fat out of the body.
+ **Garlic** helps lower cholesterol and helps in detoxification.
+ **Chromium Picolinate**, a trace mineral, aids with burning fat and reducing sugar cravings.
+ **Kelp** helps support the thyroid and assists the metabolism in utilizing energy.
+ **Peppermint Leaf** tea decreases appetite.
+ **Chickweed** helps reduce appetite.
+ **Bladderwrack**, a sea vegetable, enhances energy.

These supplements function as a weight-loss tonic by building energy, suppressing appetite, burning fat, aiding digestion, and/or acting as a diuretic.

Heart Disease

+ **Alfalfa** decreases blood cholesterol and adds minerals.
+ **Parsley** acts as a diuretic.
+ **Gingko Biloba** improves circulation and getting oxygen to all cells.
+ **Vitamin E** helps protect estrogen in the body and slows hardening of the arteries.
+ **Mandrake Root** lowers high blood pressure and strengthens the heart.

+ **Motherwort** has sedative effects and reduces heart rate.
+ **Hawthorne Berry** improves the blood supply to the heart.
+ **Magnesium** and **potassium** help regulate the heartbeat.
+ **Vitamin B-6** prevents blood clots and lowers cholesterol.
+ **Vitamin C** strengthens blood vessels and keeps plaque from building on the walls of the arteries.
+ **Co-enzyme Q-10** prevents damage to the heart and helps oxygenate the blood.

These substances work together and assist the body in improving circulation and lowering cholesterol and blood pressure.

Diabetes

+ **Chromium** improves glucose tolerance and increases insulin levels.
+ **Potassium** improves glucose metabolism.
+ **Vitamin B** complex lowers the need for insulin and detoxifies stress.
+ **Dandelion** assists and supports the pancreas.
+ **Fenugreek** is known as a blood sugar-lowering herb.
+ **Blueberry** acts like insulin in the body and is less toxic.
+ **Bilberry** helps the body eliminate excess glucose.

These herbs assist the body in assimilating nutrients and help support the pancreas and lower blood-sugar levels.

CHINESE MEDICINE

The Chinese are known for their two-thousand-year-old use of traditional Chinese medicine. They believe disease is caused by disharmony. The treatment tools consist of diet, herbs, acupuncture, exercise, and meditation, which helps us overcome illness by neutralizing disharmony by treating the mind, body, and spirit. The disharmony and discomforts we experience during menopause are positively impacted by the strategies inherent in the practice of Chinese medicine. The philosophy is based on maintaining wholeness, restoring harmony, and the prevention of illness. These are goals that every woman should strive to achieve during midlife transition.

The yin/yang concept is difficult for us to understand, but it is crucial to the way the body operates. They believe yin and yang operate as opposing forces and disease results when they are not balanced. The concept of life forces, or qi, is also central to their view of medicine as well as shen, the spirit, and jing, the nurturer of growth and development.

> **Africans were some of the first people to use herbal medicine to treat almost every ailment, according to Marcellus A. Walker, M.D. and Kenneth B. Singleton, M.D. in *Natural Health for African-Americans*. Traditional African healing focuses on seeing the body in a holistic sense and blending religion and science. Healers utilized a variety of strategies, including rituals, communication with ancestors, praying, and using plant remedies.**

My Experience with Chinese medicine

I used Chinese medicine to help me cope with my sleep disorder and am using it now to help lower my cholesterol. Hen Sen Chin, my herbalist, is eighty-two years old and has been practicing for fifty-one years. In his country, he would be considered a doctor. He told me that in his culture, people always look to food first to help them heal. Hen Sen placed me on a diet that helps my body rid itself of toxins. He says my system has too much yang (fire) and not enough yin (serenity). I had to eliminate certain foods that I had been eating frequently, such as chicken, smoked salmon, and turkey, foods I ate to take the place of red meat. He does not believe it is healthy to eat brown rice or tomatoes. According to my profile, these foods are not good for me. Chinese medicine is practiced in a way that is very specific to the needs of each individual.

Hen Sen describes my diet as bland. It includes eating white fish such as halibut, cod, perch, sole, snapper, and sea bass. I eat a variety of green vegetables, but the only pasta on the diet is a rice noodle. For breakfast I have apples, berries or pears, and hot cereal. Fruits with a lot of acid like pineapple are not allowed. Grits are also part of the plan. A bagel or English muffin with light cream cheese is allowed once per week. Brown bread is not permitted, although cornbread is. No more than two cups of coffee per day are allowed, and no soda pop or other foods that have no nutritional value. This regimen is quite similar to the macrobiotic diet, but with less consumption of grains except during winter. He believes some high-fiber foods and grains are hard for the body to digest. He says Americans eat too much meat. When he was a child, his family would be considered rich if they could have meat once a week.

I am given a large packet of herbs to make a tea and digestive pills to help my body detox. These herbs are selected from a supply of more than one thousand herbs that he orders from China. The herbs have to be put in an eight-quart glass or stainless steel pot filled to the top with spring water and cooked daily for three hours until there is only one cup of liquid left. The smell is awful, and it looks like mud. But when I follow his plan, I have high energy and mental clarity, and after several months I feel vibrant and fully alive.

Life Lesson

Healing the body takes time. The habits and practices we have developed over our lifetime cannot be fixed in a few weeks or sometimes even in a few months. Chinese medicine has taught me the beauty of patience.

ACUPUNCTURE

The purpose of acupuncture is to restore the flow of energy along the body meridians, which are points located throughout the body. Tiny needles stimulate points along meridians. The meridians correspond with certain organs and bodily functions. Once balance is restored, the body begins to heal itself. It is believed that acupuncture helps balance yin and yang while restoring the natural flow of energy through the body.

The National Center for Complementary and Alternative Medicine has documented the usefulness of acupuncture for treating a variety of conditions. It is a medical procedure that has been used for more than two thousand years and it is estimated that Americans are spending as much as $500 million per year on the procedure. There are more than eighteen thousand nationally certified acupuncturists in this country today. In World Health Organization and National Institute of Health clinical studies, acupuncture has been found to be effective for treating menopausal symptoms, blood pressure, anxiety, stress, depression, and insomnia.

HOMEOPATHY

Homeopathy is a natural system of medicine based on four basic premises. The first one is that like cures like. The second is that the therapy attempts to bring out the vital forces of the body to cure itself and does not focus on suppressing symptoms. The third is that only a single remedy is needed, and the fourth premise states that a minimal dosage is required. Homeopaths use small portions of plants or minerals to stimulate the body's healing mechanism. These remedies help the body heal faster and they strive to correct the underlying causes of the condition. Homeopaths do not believe in disease so much as they believe that symptoms are a manifestation of things happening outside of normal functioning for a particular individual. Every condition is seen as unique to the individual because of each person's personality, character, emotional makeup, heredity, diet, life circumstances, environment, and the way they respond to the disease. They believe that each patient must be educated about living a healthy lifestyle and must understand how to promote health.

What a person experiences on the mental level is considered to be most important. You need to be prepared to talk about your feelings when you consult a homeopath. Homeopaths believe all healing starts on the inside and moves to the outside. When the psychological symptoms decrease, the physical symptoms intensify and a cure is often imminent. The laws of homeopathic medicine state that symptoms disappear in the reverse order from the way they appeared. Once healing begins, some symptoms can reappear, and in many cases symptoms manifest in the upper body and then move to the lower body. General symptoms are felt throughout the body and are not limited to one body part, like particular symptoms.

Samuel Hahnemann, a German doctor, discovered the principles of this system of medicine in 1790. He conducted "provings" on healthy individuals and felt strongly that the body is capable of healing itself and that physicians should be led by observation and experience to treat the person and not the symptoms. He studied chronic as well as acute illnesses to develop his methods and was considered to be very radical because he didn't subscribe to popular medical practices.

Hahnemann stated, "Since diseases are only deviations from the healthy condition and since they express themselves through symptoms, and since cure is equally only a change from the diseased condition back to the state of health, one sees that medicines can cure disease only if they possess the power to alter the way a person feels and functions." He believed in a holistic approach to medicine and was committed to finding ways to improve physical and spiritual well-being.

Because homeopathic remedies encompass the mental, physical, and emotional aspects of a condition or illness, they should be beneficial in treating symptoms of menopause such as hot flashes and other symptoms that are often recurring and are tied to our mental and physical well-being. When you consult with a qualified homeopathic professional, take a journal of your symptoms noting severity, time of onset, and the sensations tied to each symptom. Be prepared to speak in great detail about what you are experiencing.

Your homeopathic practitioner will want to know things like:

◆ What makes the symptoms worse?
◆ What makes the symptoms better?
◆ What was happening to you when you first noted it?
◆ How did it make you feel?
◆ How did you behave and how is this symptom different from what is normal for you?
◆ How often has it occurred?
◆ Does it affect more than one part of your body?

Homeopaths assess your overall level of health and your lifestyle barriers to optimal health, such as poor nutrition, lack of exercise, negative relationships, self-defeating attitudes, too much stress, and poor quality of life. The remedy will closely match your symptoms and involve a more intuitive approach than what you might expect.

There are a wide variety of homeopathic remedies; approximately two thousand are known today. Many are made from plants, minerals, chemical substances, and exotic substances like pickled spider. Other homeopathic remedies are made from common substances, like oyster shells, red onions, and chocolate.

Homeopathic remedies for menopausal symptoms include:

♦ **Sepia.** Sepia is helpful for fatigue, low moods, sweating, and mood swings. It is made from a fluid found in the body of cuttlefish.

♦ **Sanguinaria.** This remedy is useful during perimenopause for symptoms of heavy flow during menstruation and headaches. It is also recommended for night sweats and breast tenderness, and for a person who is often anxious. This root comes from a plant in the poppy family and is a native plant of North America.

♦ **Cimicifuga racemosa.** Cimicifuga is an herb made from dried roots. It is a perennial plant and is also known as black cohosh or black snakeroot. It is effective for the treatment of depression at menopause. It is usually prescribed for people who are emotionally sensitive and has been used by Native Americans for a long time.

♦ **Causticum.** Causticum is used to treat sleep disturbances, emotional stress and anxiety. It is also helpful for people who are mentally fatigued. This remedy is made of slaked lime, also known as calcium hydroxide, and potassium bisulphate, and is based on a formula proven by Hahnemann.

AYURVEDIC MEDICINE

Ayurvedic medicine is a system of healing from India that has been around for more than three thousand years. According to the *Gale Encyclopedia of Alternative Medicine,* it is known as the science of living a long and healthy life. Ayurveda is preventative and also serves to correct imbalances. It is often used in this country to complement traditional medicine. It focuses on locating and treating the root causes of diseases and treats them with healing strategies including detoxification, cleansing, meditation, herbal remedies, massage therapy, and yoga. According to Ayurvedic medicine, the body is seen as composed of doshas, or body types. Each individual has a unique blend of the three doshas: kapha, pitta, and vata. Disease occurs when we develop imbalances in one or more dosha.

Deepak Chopra, M.D., a leading authority on Ayurvedic medicine, has written several books describing the techniques and how they can be used to treat a variety of conditions including high blood pressure, obesity, depression, diabetes, and heart disease, conditions that many African-American women are facing.

Susan McKinney Steward, M.D., was the first Black woman to practice medicine in New York State. She obtained her degree in 1870 from the New York Medical College for Women, a homeopathic medical school, and graduated as valedictorian of her class. African-American physicians in the New York area have named their medical society the Susan McKinney Steward Medical Society to honor her.

NATIVE AMERICAN MEDICINE

The Native Americans in this country have a long history of using herbs and natural medicine. Native Americans have great respect for nature and the future of this planet. They view all plants as natural resources. As early as the middle 1600s, Native Americans used echinacea and ginseng. Their medicine has been studied by anthropologists and categorized as ethnomedicine, the healing practices of native cultures.

To learn more about Native American medicine, I have had several meetings with Alice Micco Snow, herbalist for the Seminole Tribe of Florida and coauthor of *Healing Plants.* She is not a Native American doctor, but a collector of herbs. She also acts as a go-between for the doctor and the patient. She wrote her book to help capture and document traditional Native American medicine so that her people would not lose this knowledge and important part of their culture. Alice Snow recognizes about seventy-five different herbs by sight. There are several plants used to treat women's conditions, including menopause, heart problems, stroke, and hysterectomy. There are two hundred herbs used by Native Americans in the southeastern United States and most grow in their immediate environment, but they will also travel to neighboring states to collect certain herbs, according to Alice. The Seminole doctors sing over the herbs because they believe this gives them more power. The treatments are used for prevention and healing throughout the life cycle, including midlife transition.

Developing Nutritional Strategies

We must learn to develop positive and healthy life patterns without feeling that our cultural identity is being attacked. Our people practiced positive eating habits, such as eating lots of vegetables, especially our traditional collard greens and okra, which are very healthy when cooked without a lot of fat. Traditionally, we have always eaten whole foods, such as grains, corn, sweet potatoes, and yams.

As we celebrate our strengths and the things we do well, we should become more cognizant of the patterns we need to eliminate. I don't mean to imply that all our food habits are based on negative patterns, because it is clear our ancestors established a variety of good patterns of wellness behavior that we have neglected to follow. But over the past thirty years, we have begun to eat more like other Americans who are consuming fast food like it is going out of style.

Looking back on conversations with the elders in my family, I recall that they did not eat fast food. They did not consider a hamburger and fries as a "real meal." Whenever we go to Memphis to visit relatives, they cook enough food for an army and everything is cooked traditionally. Of course, some of the food has too much fat, like our traditional greens with pork ham hocks, but other dishes are quite healthy. Today, all of us have begun to incorporate healthier ways of seasoning food, such as using smoked turkey parts in our greens and cutting down on the amount of pork we consume. It is rare these days for any of us to eat fried foods. What is your family doing to eat better?

My grandmother insisted on at least three vegetables with lunch and dinner. A meal was not complete without serving sliced cucumbers and tomatoes. She also didn't believe in eating late. Going to bed early was a longtime habit, and she got plenty of exercise because she didn't believe in sitting down for more than a few moments. Living on a farm in rural Mississippi gave her plenty of opportunities for daily exercise.

Healthy foods that have been widely used in Africa:
♦ Corn
♦ Millet
♦ Lentils
♦ Chickpeas
♦ Yams/sweet potatoes
♦ Okra
♦ Black-eyed peas
♦ Red beans

Understanding our cultural beliefs about food and exercise is a good place to start as we strive to be well. As you know, in our culture, good food is often a very important part of every major celebration. In my family, my cousins and I made a commitment to break the pattern of obesity, high blood pressure, and bad health that had plagued my family for generations. It is up to all of us to develop innovative programs and healthy diets. This commitment will have a positive effect on our families and our communities.

STRATEGIES FOR DEVELOPING GOOD EATING HABITS
Prepare a weekly menu

One of the most important methods for developing good eating habits is to prepare your meals in advance. When I start a week without a clue about what I intend to eat, I end up consuming a lot of junk. Since I don't like to cook, I have to be innovative about having my husband cook for me before he leaves town, buying low-fat deli meals, or preparing one large item to eat for several days. Sometimes I eat lots of leftovers, but it works for me.

Hire someone to cook for you

I have used several different cooking services where they come to my home and fix ten to twelve meals, label them, and put them in the freezer, or they cook the food and deliver meals twice a month. I had to fill out a questionnaire and state my preferences, and I always select services that provided a wide variety of low-fat meals. Some of my friends assumed that the cooking services were expensive, but were surprised when I told them that you end up paying about $10 per serving or less. The time factor is important too. Many of us don't feel we have enough time to cook, and find ourselves grabbing fast, convenient, and often unhealthy food. It is an investment in your health. We have to make the commitment to do whatever it takes to get healthy.

Each meal is designed for two servings, but depending on the dish, I found that many dishes lasted for three or more servings. In the long run, I saved money on food because my grocery shopping consisted of buying fruit, juice, and cereal. This is a good option because the meals are ready to eat with minimal preparation and you know exactly how many calories and how much fat you're consuming.

Forget about fad diets

I have tried all types of fad diets, but I don't bother anymore because I know they don't work. I have also tried a lot of the natural products that are guaranteed to help you burn fat faster and suppress your appetite. Using these supplements was my way of trying to find a quick fix. But when it comes to weight control and healthy eating, we know there is no such thing.

Change your thinking about food

I learned that I had to change my mindset about eating adequate fruits and vegetables. I visualize all the antioxidants and beta carotene that I'm packing in to prevent cancer cells from developing in my body. I was raised eating vegetables that were often overcooked and heavily seasoned. I didn't care much for them. Once I realized that I prefer my vegetables lightly steamed and delicately seasoned with fresh herbs like basil, thyme, and rosemary, I began to eat more of them. This is another one of those cultural things you may have experienced as well. My parents cooked vegetables the way they were used to eating them. Many African-Americans were raised eating this way and we were taught to clean our plates whether we were hungry or not.

The human body is a complex organism that depends on many factors to keep it thriving and working properly. We need to be more aware of the nutrients required to make our bodies work the way they were designed to work. Protein, essential fatty acids, carbohydrates, minerals, and vitamins all serve a purpose and work together in a delicate and synchronized fashion. When one component is missing, it throws everything off. As we get older, we begin to pay a heavy price for not understanding how our bodies work. As always, our belief systems play a significant role. We often eat what we have been conditioned to eat.

What impacts our beliefs about what we eat?

- **Our culture**: the way we see the world and what we consider to be normal
- **Our environment**: what we see happening around us and the food readily available
- **Schools**: what we were served and were used to eating for most of our childhood
- **Family**: the eating habits of our parents and relatives, how we celebrated holidays and cultural events
- **Society**: what society teaches us about food and the foods we are encouraged to eat through media exposure
- **Religion**: some foods have religious connotations and are forbidden by religious doctrine

During menopause, many of our bad habits start to exact a higher price. Ann Louise Gittleman, author of *Supernutrition for Menopause,* theorizes that our greatest challenge is not that our ovaries stop producing estrogen but that our adrenal glands are depleted by poor lifestyle habits. The adrenal glands are the estrogen backup system and should start producing more estrogen and progesterone as our ovaries produce less. She believes the detrimental effects of eating too much caffeine and sugar and not enough of essential fatty acids like omega-3 (fish oil) and flax seed oil lead to a state where our adrenal system fails to function properly. The consequences of this scenario increase our risk of heart disease, diabetes, and osteoporosis. She states, "Menopause can be a positive motivational factor to make the dietary and lifestyle changes that will ease not only our passage through menopause, but benefit our health for the rest of our lives."

WHAT'S SOY GOT TO DO WITH IT?

There are certain foods that contain phytoestrogens or plant estrogens, including soy. When consumed, they can reduce menopause symptoms such as hot flashes and irritability. Dr. Klein at the University of Illinois has studied the effect of soy on menopause symptoms, especially hot flashes. Over several years, she implemented a breakfast club where menopausal women came in several mornings per week to practice preparing and tasting various soy recipes. They made muffins and breads using granulated soy. All of the soy was ordered from the same source. Some of the women were on estrogen, and some consumed 44 mg of soy each day. A significant number of the women who experienced mild symptoms alleviated them by eating soy.

Women who consume diets high in soy have a reduced risk of cancer. The World Health Organization rates Japanese women as the healthiest people in the Second Half of Life. This has been attributed to eating as much as 30 mg of soy daily as well as other lifestyle factors, including eating smaller portions of dairy products, meat, and sugar. Eating soy products can help us African-American women reduce cholesterol and positively impact our high rates of heart disease.

More research needs to be done to document the impact of soy on the health of African-Americans. However, preliminary studies indicate that it may be quite beneficial.

MIDLIFE NUTRITIONAL TIPS

Although I believe in eating less meat, women on a vegetarian diet tend to have difficulty getting adequate, high-quality protein. Deficiency in these areas can lead to early menopause because the pituitary glands and ovaries may not be getting the necessary support. To help delay menopause, women need eggs, fish, yogurt, lots of vegetables, grains, legumes, and nuts. Foods with B complex, such as brewer's yeast, omega fish oils, flax seed, and evening primrose oil are recommended.

SEVEN-DAY FOOD PLAN FOR AFRICAN-AMERICAN WOMEN IN MENOPAUSE
Breakfast Choices
* Oat cereal with melon and yogurt
* Egg-white omelet with vegetables, cantaloupe, and wheat toast
* Low-fat cottage cheese, wheat cereal, and twelve-grain toast with spreadable fruit
* Low-fat granola, wheat bagel with low-fat cream cheese
* Turkey sausage with sliced tomatoes and melba toast

Lunch choices
* Spinach salad with fresh crabmeat
* Tuna with celery and low-fat mayo on rye bread, cup of veggie soup
* Chicken breast wrap with carrot sticks
* Veggie burger in wheat pita with salsa and shredded lettuce
* Low-fat shrimp gumbo with fat-free crackers
* Chef salad with low-fat dressing and egg drop soup

Dinner choices
* Broiled catfish with steamed broccoli and corn on the cob
* Chili with ground turkey, low-fat corn bread, and collard greens seasoned with turkey parts
* Oven-baked chicken breast with corn flake breading and mustard greens with sliced tomatoes
* Stuffed cabbage with ground turkey and peas and couscous
* Dirty rice with red kidney beans, steamed okra, and a small green salad
* Seafood stir-fry with soba noodles, scallops, bean sprouts, and bok choy

♦ Shrimp scampi with wild rice and asparagus (grilled with sunflower oil or olive oil)

Snacks
- Grapes, berries, and watermelon
- Roasted soy nuts
- Bagel chips and salsa
- Salt-free wheat pretzels
- Soy milk smoothie with banana
- Sunflower seeds

Supplements for menopause
♦ Calcium, 1500 mg (builds strong bones)
♦ B complex, 100 mg (helps with menopause low moods, improves energy level and hormone balance, counteracts stress)
♦ Vitamin C, 3000 mg (boosts immune system)
♦ Linseed oil, 4 capsules (helps prevent cardiovascular disease and coronary heart disease)
♦ Vit E, 800 I.U. (fights free radicals and relieves hot flashes)
♦ Selenium, 200 mcg (reduces cancer risk)
♦ L-Carnitine, 500 mg (an amino acid that assists in weight loss and heart disease)
♦ Zinc, 100 mg (beneficial for healthy hair, skin, and nails)
♦ Magnesium, 750 mg (helps with insomnia, anxiety, and muscle cramps)
♦ Vitamin A, 20,000 IU (reduces cancer risk, helps with vision, boosts immune system, and promotes healthy skin)

HEALTHY EATING TIPS

- Avoid smoked foods.
- Buy fresh vegetables.
- Look for low-sodium products.
- Flavor your food with fresh herbs.
- Taste your food before adding salt.
- Avoid canned or processed foods.
- Read labels for hidden ingredients and preservatives.
- Reduce fat and protein.
- Make sure that you get phosphorous, but not so much that it neutralizes calcium.
- Eat lots of collard greens (very high in calcium). One cup has 357 mg of calcium.
- Minimize carbonated beverages.
- Increase calcium-rich foods.

EAT PHYTOESTROGENS

Eating plants that mimic estrogen in the body can help relieve some of your symptoms during menopause. These plants are called phytoestrogens. Practically every plant has some type of substance that is similar to estrogen.

Foods high in phytoestrogens include fruits, vegetables (greens, spinach, and cabbage, which are often eaten by African-Americans), soy, flaxseed, sprouts, and beans (especially peas and lentils).

NUTRITION TIPS FOR MOOD DISORDERS

Serotonin-rich foods help with low moods:

- Corn, wild rice, oats, brown rice, wheat, millet
- Whole-grain breads, bagels, tortillas, taco shells, and pasta

- Vegetables, squash (acorn, butternut, pumpkins, zucchini)
- Root vegetables and complex carbohydrates such as potatoes, turnips, yams, carrots, onions, celery, ginger

RAW FOOD DIET

This diet consists of eating fruits, vegetables, seeds, nuts, sprouts, and whole grains. It avoids cooking food, which often diminishes nutritional value by destroying or altering the vitamins, minerals, and enzymes in what we eat. Meat, dairy products, and coffee are not allowed. It sounds quite restrictive, but once you begin experimenting, you will find there are so many varieties of food to eat.

The number of raw-food enthusiasts is growing rapidly. There are self-help groups devoted to eating this way. I first became aware of them by joining in on a chat room. I went on the diet for thirty days and found it to be beneficial in many ways. My energy level increased, my complexion cleared, I lost weight, and I felt vibrant after the first ten days. I recommend it as a technique for detoxifying your body rather than as a lifelong commitment and suggest you try to incorporate more raw foods in your daily diet. It's quite clear that eating more fresh fruits and vegetables improves our health. Eating a raw-food diet for a few days or a few weeks has helped me reduce my cravings for sugar and fats.

MACROBIOTIC EATING

Macrobiotic eating is a diet I highly recommend for African-American women in menopause. According to *The Macrobiotic Way* by Michio Kushi, macrobiotic dining is based on eating whole foods, including grains, vegetables, nuts, beans, white fish, and fruit. This diet incorporates many principles of food that were popular with our ancestors in Africa and earlier generations of African-Americans in this country. Eating large amounts of grains, fruits, and vegetables is a way of life for most African and Third World people.

Macrobiotic diet in a nutshell

- **Vegetables:** broccoli, bok choy, Brussels sprouts, carrots, Chinese cabbage, greens, onions, squash, daikon greens, leeks, scallions
- **Sea vegetables:** wakame, agar, kelp, dulse, hijiki, nori, kombu
- **Grains:** whole barley, buckwheat, corn, brown rice, whole rye, oats, and other whole grains
- **Beans:** aduki, chickpeas, lentils, miso natto (soybeans), tempeh, tofu bean curd (eat a limited amount; no more than 10 percent of food consumption)
- **Fish:** white fish, flounder, haddock, halibut, herring, smelt, sole, trout
- **Fruits:** watermelon, grapes, apples, peaches, plums, pears, prunes, tangerines, apricots, berries, cherries, cantaloupe, dried fruits (should be 10 percent or less of daily food consumption)
- **Sweeteners:** apple juice or cider, rice malt, rice syrup
- **Condiments:** Tamari soy sauce, sea salt, kelp, sesame salt, ginger, brown rice vinegar, pickled vegetables
- **Teas:** Amasake tea, bancha green tea, roasted barley tea, rice tea
- **Snacks:** pumpkin seeds, sunflower seeds, rice cakes, almonds, peanuts
- **Oils:** brown sesame oil or unrefined corn oil; olive oil is OK occasionally
- **Beverages:** Avoid coffee and drink spring or well water

Proportions of the macrobiotic diet

50–60 percent whole grains and products made from grains
20–30 percent vegetables
5–10 percent beans and sea vegetables and soups
5 percent complementary foods, condiments, fish, and beverages

Advantages of the macrobiotic food plan for African-American women

Most of us eat a diet that is fiber-deficient, which leads to diseases of the digestive system. This diet provides a healthy amount of fiber. Fiber is the part of a plant that provides the structure. It moves through our bodies without changing much and adds necessary bulk. Research shows that in African countries where the people eat high-fiber diets, they are 80 percent less likely to develop colon cancer. But African-Americans in the United States develop colon cancer at the same rate as the rest of the country. Colon cancer is the third-ranking cause of death in the United States.

MENOPAUSE CALL TO ACTION

- Use complementary medicine to help you take charge of your health during perimenopause and menopause.
- Change your eating habits by applying your increased knowledge about nutrition, vitamin supplementation, and the importance of physical fitness.
- Commit to reducing your risks of developing the "big three" for African-American women: heart disease, diabetes, and high blood pressure.
- Manage stress and immerse yourself in applying information about the mind/body connection.
- Enhance your vital force through principles of Chinese medicine and Ayervedic medicine.
- Incorporate the best of our African ancestry in the way you live your life today.
- Get started now!

PERSONAL SUCCESS HEALTH PLAN

Make a commitment in the following areas as needed:

♦ Exercise

♦ Change your eating habits

♦ Lose weight

♦ Take time for leisure activities and hobbies

♦ Pamper yourself

♦ Incorporate preventive and complementary medicine principles in your life

♦ Sample low-fat cooking recipes

Sign your name to this plan and keep it posted where you can see it. Change the plan every few months as needed.

I, _____, am fully committed to improving my health at midlife. I sign this contract to remind me of my responsibility and commitment to improve my health, mentally, spiritually, and physically.

Date: _____

Witness: _____

Ask a friend or someone from your sister network to witness the contract and act as a mentor or buddy to help you remember your plan.

CHAPTER 10

Share Your Passage with Your Sisters

Openly sharing perimenopause and menopause with our sisters is an empowering strategy for doing our transition differently. After mastering steps one through six of this book, it is time for the celebrations to begin. Celebrate your uniqueness. Celebrate your ability to lead a joyous life. Celebrate your longevity and loving spirit. Sisters, we have so much to feel good about in our lives.

In almost every society there are ceremonies and celebrations for each new phase of life. Our West African brothers and sisters have numerous ceremonies and rituals, including celebrations of the harvest, naming children, and celebrating their ancestors. The entire village participates and sometimes an entire region celebrates together to affirm their sense of community and spiritual connection. Rituals are performed along with storytelling, dancing, feasting, and wearing costumes. All these activities play a part in cultural extravaganzas and each component has a special meaning.

In African cultures, opening ceremonial greetings are important as a sign of welcome and respect. The initial phase of the celebration sets the tone and there is a great deal of time spent planning the opening ceremony. Music plays an important role, and every special occasion has its own type of music. Women's gatherings and ceremonies have their own music and pageantry as well.

In our culture, we don't have any ceremonies to celebrate the phases of women's lives. Most of us didn't celebrate the beginning of menstruation unless we had a progressive mother like Dr. Gwendolyn Goldsby Grant, the well-known *Essence* columnist. She says her mom created a special commemoration for her and told her she was entering womanhood. No one talked to us about womanhood and becoming our own person when we turned twenty-one. To make matters worse, women beginning menopause in our culture have had to hide their symptoms and deal with feelings of shame.

African-American women have become a little more open about discussing our menopause experiences and what happens to us at midlife. We can take it a step farther by developing supportive sister networks, using rituals to celebrate our transition, and designing our own woman-centered Afrocentric ceremonies and activities to commemorate our passage together. Talking and sharing helps us to relieve our tensions and put things in perspective. In my Do Menopause with An Attitude group, we did not develop a ritual. We are quite informal and still in the process of determining what we want to do, but I encourage you to invent a more formal way to document this right of passage. Our groups and gatherings serve many purposes.

Menopause groups do the following for us:

- Provide a place to share feelings with women who are experiencing some of the same challenges
- Provide the opportunity to break down the barriers between Black women based on age, education, economic status, sexual orientation, marital status, and skin tone
- Gives us precious time in a setting with our sisters exploring roles and our changing expectations about our lives

- Gives us a space where we reinforce our personal and spiritual growth
- Offers us a chance to talk about life lessons learned and share our collective wisdom
- Document the commonalities of our experiences even when our lifestyle choices are different

WHAT DOES SISTERHOOD REPRESENT FOR YOU?

For me, it represents being with girlfriends from the old neighborhood and my college days and sharing my feelings with women who really know all my strengths and insecurities. For the Black women I have met later in life, sisterhood represents the opportunity to share my life experiences with women who may be experiencing many of the same challenges. For my white friends, it gives me a chance to communicate cross-culturally with women with whom I have tremendous rapport and to affirm that in many ways we are more alike than different.

How do you hook up with sisters at this time in your life? There are so many groups and organizations where Black women come together, including:

- Social clubs
- Sororities
- Extended family gatherings
- Traditional African-American organizations like the Urban League and NAACP
- Church
- Neighborhood organizations
- School-related groups
- Professional organizations
- Advocacy groups

> **"Talking with one another is loving one another."**
> —*Kenyan proverb*

You can also celebrate midlife by getting involved in a cause that excites you. Make time to volunteer for a project where you can make a difference. This will help you have balance in your life. I found myself wanting to fight for a cause that would help women receive better health care. Barbara Levy is a founding board member and invited me to become a founding member of the American College of Women's Health Physicians/ Foundation for Women's Health. The goal of this organization is to get women's health certified as its own medical specialty. This would ensure that women in the future are treated by physicians who are women's health specialists, not by an OB/GYN, family practice physician, or an internist. Also, these specialists would receive comprehensive training in medical school and throughout their residency on treating the special needs of the whole woman. We have participated in several fund-raising events and community-education activities designed to help mobilize women about the need for holistic and woman-centered health-care systems. Being involved with this organization at the beginning of my transition meant a great deal to me.

I received a grant from the Speaking with An Active Voice Campaign in October of 2001 to develop a series of workshops and brown bag lunches for low-income African-American women. This was a project that provided me with the opportunity to create a community service. The American Medical Women's Association and Pharmacia Corporation granted money to fifteen women across the country to assist each of us in making a difference through our pet projects. I have met some wonderful women who would otherwise have little access to accurate information about planning for perimenopause/menopause. This work excites me and is close to my heart. I am committed to making sure these women have the latest information so they can make informed decisions about how to cope with their symptoms and the changes they face.

Barbara Levy is also involved with another exciting cause. She is one of the founders of a nonprofit group called Real Women. They are dedicated to helping women and young girls learn to love their bodies. They use storytelling and body image workshops to reach women. Dr. Levy commissioned a group of statues of nude women from ages four to eighty-four whose bodies are beautiful but not perfect. Viewing the statues is heartwarming, because you know it takes a lot of courage to expose your body with all its imperfections. The statues are on exhibit in her office and are part of a national exhibit traveling to major cities under the National Science Foundation Women's Health Exhibit.

Educating ourselves about how we are impacted by negative external forces is a big job. We have to eliminate any baggage caused by the negative historical views of women. Some of these beliefs are ingrained or internalized without our awareness. In Victorian times, it was believed women were likely to be hysterical. The word "hysterical" comes from the word "hysteria," which is derived from the Greek word "uterus." People believed that women had an intellectual capacity limited to only domestic matters, while at the same time women were supposed to be compassionate, industrious, faithful, wise, and virtuous.

In many cultures—even today—circumcisions of female genitalia are performed as well as infibulation, which is the removal of the outer genitalia and clitoris and closing of the outer parts with sutures, or, in some cases, thorns, leaving only two small openings for menstruation and urination.

These procedures fostered the belief that the female genitalia is ugly and disgusting and that women should not be free to enjoy sex. Circumcision and infibulation were not only practiced in Africa, but also in Western Europe and America in the nineteenth century for little girls who were caught masturbating. Up until 1935, American hospitals practiced circumcision as a cure for melancholy or depression, masturbation, and epilepsy. This abuse was rationalized by the belief that women are inferior and a menace to men because we tempt them to sin.

How much of these feelings of inferiority still reside in our subconscious, only to be aggravated by menopause? If we still believe on some level that we must be humiliated, then menopause becomes one more passage where we allow ourselves to be victimized by the way others perceive the natural development of our bodies. It doesn't make sense to be ashamed of our biology. What views have you inherited along with menopause? What myths, collective thinking, stereotypes, and misconceptions? Some of us are plagued by erroneous beliefs that tell us older women are over the hill. Sharing our stories helps us validate our power.

Did you know...

Did you know in many cultures menopause is a rite of passage to greater power?

Did you know women in India are only allowed to talk and interact in certain social situations with men after menopause?

Did you know women in Ethiopia are invited to participate in ceremonies and walk on sacred ground after menopause?

Did you know in many Native American tribes women are seen as wise and spiritually gifted after going thirteen months with no period?

Menopause is a time to follow your bliss. But first we have to believe we're worthy of it. Then we have to know what bliss is for us.

This is a time to check out your relationships with the women in your life. Do you have a supportive network? Who can you talk to about what's happening to you and how you feel about it? Did you know there is a connection between good health and emotional support?

Spending more time with other women during menopause has enhanced my life and made my midlife transition easier. I have spent more time talking with both of my sisters, my mom, and my friends. We have always discussed everything but now we also talk about aging with grace. We discuss our goals in achieving optimal health and fitness. Sharing your perimenopause/menopause transition with other women enhances the experience. It is another passage in life that requires the emotional support and camaraderie of friendship.

> **"Communal bonds forged by shared historical, cultural, and spiritual experiences have made us family."**
>
> —*Joan Morgan*

Some of us may have limited knowledge about our mothers' transition. This is unfortunate, but it is often difficult for African-American mothers to share the details of their transition. They entered menopause at a different time. If possible, talk with as many women in your family as possible so you have more information about your menopausal family history. Sharing across the generations helps us document our feminine family legacy.

AFFIRMATIONS

- Sharing my journey with my "sistahs" rekindles my faith in the goodness of life.
- At midlife, I share my wisdom and knowledge joyfully with other women.
- I choose to be happy at midlife and I talk about my journey.
- Midlife is a great adventure and I take pride in the beauty of my transformation.
- The company of my sisters during menopause sustains me.

Life Lesson

Whether we feel anger, sadness, or frustration, we have stop to hiding and repressing our feelings. Menopause is a good time to get things out in the open and to work on letting go. We need to be kinder to ourselves and nurture our softer side. As Black women making our way in this country, we have often been forced to be harsh in order to survive. Perhaps we have earned the right to let our guard down and be honest with ourselves and with others about how we really feel inside.

MENOPAUSE ROLE MODELS

There are several women who come to mind immediately when I think of menopause role models for us. Cecily Tyson is in her sixties, but she is still the epitome of elegance and self-confidence.

Camille Cosby is another woman who is strong, beautiful, and elegant. She has weathered a great tragedy with the death of her only son but continues to be a strong role model. I could probably list a hundred women who are well-known, over fifty, and are leading fabulous lives and making great contributions to society.

> **"Any woman can look her best if she feels good in her skin. It's not a question of clothes or makeup. It's how she sparkles."**
> —*Sophia Loren*

I can't wait to see how a free spirit like Whoopi Goldberg will handle her transition. Who do you think of as strong and wise African-American women in midlife? What about selecting historical mentors from the likes of Sojourner Truth, bell hooks, Audre Lourde, Mary McCleod Bethune, Zora Neale Hurston, and Harriet Tubman? For more contemporary choices, what about Joycelyn Elders, Dr. Vivian Pinn, Ruby Dee, Lena Horne, Oprah Winfrey, Patti LaBelle,

Johnetta Cole, Ruth Simmons, and Alexis Herman? What is their legacy to us?

There's a multitude of Black women who are making a contribution to the world. There are also many ordinary Black women doing extraordinary things. Looking at them helps to reaffirm that we have a great deal to look forward to.

"If an eagle waited for perfect conditions, it would never soar," said Byrd Bagget in *Dare to Soar*. "We must have the courage to bet on our dreams, to take the calculated risk and leave behind forever the internal forces that hold us down."

> **"If you have a purpose in which you can believe, there's no end to the amount of things you can accomplish."**
> —*Marian Anderson*

I find conditions are never perfect for taking charge of your health and your future. But inspirational quotes and stories help me focus and develop my own personal mission statement. At different stages of my life I have had different mission statements, always tied to my desire to help others and continue my own pursuit of personal excellence. My current mission is to empower myself and other African-American women to take charge of our health care and celebrate the Second Half of our lives.

WRITING A PERSONAL MISSION STATEMENT

A personal mission statement gives us a track on which to run our lives. Just like a train track guides the direction of the train, our version of who we are and what we stand for gives us a path to follow. A personal mission statement serves this purpose in our lives and is a blueprint for the future. It describes our purpose, our passion, and the tasks we are called upon to accomplish.

The process of writing helps you clarify, fine-tune, and guide your actions. Each new challenge is assessed on the basis of how it fits with your guiding principles, which must be established before you can write an effective mission statement. Sharing your mission statement with other women opens up discussions about life and can lead to some fantastic conversations.

Answer the following questions:

♦ What are my priorities?

♦ What values or principles represent my purpose in midlife?

Select words that describe your values, words like "honesty," "caring," "respect," "character," "integrity," and "compassion". Use these words to talk about your general aim and purpose at this stage of your life.

Marian Wright Edelman said, "The legacy I want to leave is a child-care system that says no kid is going to be left alone or unsafe."

Mary McCleod Bethune said, "Invest in the human soul. Who knows, it might be a diamond in the rough."

We've all heard about Kwanzaa celebrations. The Kwanzaa tradition developed by Maulana Ron Karenga in 1966 has become a popular way for African-Americans to celebrate the holiday season in a way that affirms our culture and our sense of purpose. The seven principles are unity, faith, self-determination, collective work, purpose, cooperative economics, and creativity. The principles involved represent the type of themes you might consider incorporating in your personal mission statement. Use ideas that inspire you to take action.

Achieving our mission in life is our legacy. It's tied to our sense of purpose. It reminds us of what we're meant to do. When we are operating based on our mission statement, it motivates us to move forward. At midlife, we have more psychological tools and mental fortitude to achieve our true purpose.

Using a mission statement to keep us "in check" also helps us avoid getting in a rut. You may be in a mental rut and used to thinking the same way about your life events. If you are in a rut in any area of your life, get your group members to help you climb out and then put together an action plan for moving forward.

How do you know when you're in a rut?
♦ A lack of excitement about life
♦ No positive expectancy of the future
♦ Feeling like you're not growing
♦ A sense of restlessness or boredom
♦ You move through life without having to think

How do you jump out of a rut?
♦ Use your imagination.
♦ Look at where you want to be and focus on what you want.
♦ Don't second-guess yourself.
♦ Take action.
♦ Use your intuition to figure out what's best for you.
♦ Get rid of your mental barriers to success.

AFRICAN-AMERICAN WOMEN FULFILLING THEIR PURPOSE IN LIFE
Dr. Shawne Bryant

Two years ago, I had the opportunity to interview Dr. Shawne Bryant, an OB/GYN physician practicing in Virginia Beach. She strikes me as a woman who is truly living her purpose in life. She encourages her patients to take a holistic approach to health at midlife and she also incorporates strategies in traditional and nontraditional medicine in her practice. As a licensed massage therapist, she gives her patients massages as part of their treatment. She believes woman-centered health care is more than taking care of a woman's reproductive system. She believes she must educate her patients so they can educate their families about nutrition and holistic health. She is known to send her patients home with low-fat recipes, vitamins, and advice on how to manage the stresses of their lives. She also practices aromatherapy and presents workshops and wellness retreats.

Dr. Bryant's advice to women of all ages: take quiet time each day and pay attention to your bodies while replenishing your mental and spiritual health. She renews her spirit by spending time on her organic farm. She is also committed to protecting the environment and educating her community about organic fruits and vegetables.

Gwendolyn Goldsby Grant, Ph.D.

I had a fantastic conversation with Dr. Gwendolyn Goldsby Grant, columnist for *Essence* and author of *The Best Kind of Loving: A Black Woman's Guide to Finding Intimacy*. Dr. Goldsby Grant encourages us to forget about all the negative stereotypes tied to menopause and focus on feeling our power. She talked to me about how we are not defined by our physiology, but by our spirit. She speaks lovingly of the guidance and nurturing she received from her mother at every stage of her development. Her mother coached her through puberty and menopause in a way that helped her appreciate her womanhood.

In a 1998 *Essence* article on menopause, Dr. Goldsby Grant wrote, "Over 50 does not mean over the hill or scatterbrained or in the throes of a hot flash. It means that you're finally in the driver's seat, fully in charge of your life and unencumbered by the fear associated with lack of knowledge about the changes that are happening to you."

An inspiration to us all, she has a wealth of information to share on our relationships with our men. In her book, she talks about how we can't analyze our lives without looking at how our self-esteem has been shaped by our history of slavery and second-class citizenship. She comments, "Too many men and women of African descent have unwittingly bought into destructive cultural myths, with the result that we sometimes see each other as stereotypes, rather than as people."

SELF-ESTEEM AND SELF-WORTH

Since we live in a world that doesn't value age, beauty, and wisdom in older women, we must value ourselves even more. We must take responsibility for boosting our self-esteem and reinforcing the positives in our lives.

Our mothers and grandmothers didn't have choices. We do. We can make the future the next wonderful phase of our lives. Explore your history and what the women in your family did to heal themselves. We can learn a great deal about where we have come from just by listening and collecting the old stories and legends. I enjoyed a tradition of women who believed in their innate ability to thrive in the face of many challenges. That strength sustains me. I try to live according to their tradition by following my dreams, facing risks, and making a contribution. But I never forget I am fortunate to be alive during a time where I am able to assert myself and speak my mind without risking my life.

We are the first generation of Black women who can truly celebrate who we are upon reaching menopause. Menopause is a time to make sure that we become the women we want to be. It is our chance to soar! Spending quality time with other women helps us do that.

For most women, a strong need to please probably started during prehistoric times when we had a real need to be protected by our males. In Victorian times, white women were seen as property and treated like infants. African-American slave women had to please everyone. We had no rights and couldn't make any of our own decisions. But even today, we can get so caught up in pleasing our partners, our bosses, and our families, that we neglect the important women in our lives.

STARTING A DO MENOPAUSE WITH AN ATTITUDE GROUP

Many of us already have a circle of "sistah" friends, but if you're like me you may find that you neglect your circle when you get too busy, stressed out, or fall in love.

There are many ways to start a Do Menopause with An Attitude group. Gather some sisters together or reconnect with your old group and bring everyone together again. You will need to talk about how often you plan to meet. Other things to consider:

♦ Select a location for the meetings.
♦ Agree on a few guidelines about confidentiality and how to remain focused on your topics.
♦ Decide if you want to have a set agenda for each meeting or a more open format.
♦ You can contact other groups and get suggestions from them.
♦ Renew your sisterhood. We have always learned from our girl-friends, but during menopause and perimenopause, let's do it by intent.
♦ Focus on special topics or even start a Celebrate Menopause book club.
♦ Spend time gathering information about resources to help your group get focused.
♦ Plan an overnight trip to a spa or fancy hotel in your area. Use this event to jumpstart your sessions.

CELEBRATE MENOPAUSE GREETING CARDS

It is difficult to find greeting cards to send to our sisters when they begin this passage. I have developed my own. Use the following statements to design Celebrate Menopause cards and greetings:

- ♦ Don't let those flashes steal your joy. You are experiencing a summer moment.
- ♦ Girlfriend! Celebrate your passage into a bright and wonderful future.
- ♦ Welcome to the Second Half of Life.
- ♦ Black women have it going on in menopause. Rejoice in your sisterhood.

RITUALS

Design rituals for your Do Menopause with An Attitude meetings. Develop an opening ritual or greeting. Use a poem, essay, or short story. It should be something that helps to set the tone and makes everyone relax and enter into a different space mentally. It could include lighting candles or using aromatherapy. Read an African folk tale or share a story about what life was like for our great grandmothers and what we have learned from their triumphs.

> "Menopause is a universal developmental event. Understanding it as such opens the door for a wide variety of ways to share this passage with other women."
> —*Joan C. Callahan,*
> **Menopause: A Midlife Passage**

Adopt a symbol of a meaningful object like a painting or piece of African art. It could be some type of artifact or sculpture. It could also be something like an eagle, a pyramid, or gem, something that represents beauty and power. It could be a picture of an African queen like Cleopatra or Nefertiti. Some menopause groups use the symbol of the crone, goddess, or wise woman, but for us I think the image of an African queen or "diva" is more appropriate. You can also set the mood by having a piece of mud cloth present in the room.

Create a theme that resonates with everyone. A theme or motto is something that touches the heart of each group member and captures the essence of the group, possibly a theme like increasing personal power or building on the strengths of our ancestors. Maybe the words from a popular song or a phrase like Sojourner Truth's famous line, "Ain't I a woman?"

Agree upon a general format during the first meeting. Have some suggestions available or ask everyone to bring in some ideas. You might want to split up into smaller groups at the first couple of meetings and spend some time coming up with suggestions on how you want to structure your group, manage your activities, and keep records of group goal achievement. Decide how often you intend to meet and who will facilitate the meetings. It's best if group leaders rotate.

Celebrate success. Sharing success stories each week as group members achieve new goals or make progress toward making changes in their lives is important. Come up with some way to applaud when a sister shares her successes with the group. Clapping, dancing, or hugging will work. Maybe she gets to wear an African headdress for the day.

Use humor. Take time to tell funny stories or experiences related to aging. Laughter is healing and it helps us bond. Don't take menopause too seriously. I have some funny menopause posters with sayings like "I know I am post-menopausal because I don't have to call Dr. Levy every week with a new symptom. I know I am in the zone because I can wear silk blouses and underwear again and I actually get cold." It's good to have open, honest sharing, but make your meetings lively, too.

The closing ritual is just as important as the opening. Recite a poem together or hold hands and sing a joyous song. Recite an African proverb.

Say a group affirmation or read the Menopause Bill of Rights from chapter 1. Play some great music. Music has always played an important role in our culture and could be used to send everyone home on a joyous note.

It may take time to develop your rituals and pull together the props and artifacts, but don't let that keep you from getting together. The act of meeting and sharing is the most important aspect. African-American women have been meeting for hundreds of years to pray together, quilt, make baskets, and can fruits and vegetables.

There are so many perimenopause/menopause-related activities that you can participate in with your group or just with a friend. Celebrating the Second Half of Life involves participating in activities with other women, such as:

- Attend a community education workshop at a women's center or hospital on some aspects of menopause.
- Review a video on menopause (see the appendix for a list of organizations that have videos and other materials).
- Visit a women's health website and discuss current information with your group members (see appendix).
- Subscribe to a menopause newsletter (see appendix).
- Agree to take yoga, meditation, acupuncture, weight training, or low-fat cooking classes together.

It's important for us to immerse ourselves in our wonderful cultural heritage so we build our inner fortitude to neutralize the racism we face on a daily basis. According to bell hooks in *Sisters of the Yam*, increasing our sense of community helps us recover ourselves. This sister is deep. When she talks about living up to our potential, she uses the words "self-recovery" in a way that is comparative to the recovery process in the Alcoholics Anonymous twelve step program.

Twenty Ways to Celebrate Menopause:

- Learn to belly dance.
- Go on a picnic.
- Celebrate a "Diva Day" where you commemorate the accomplishments of Black women.
- Have a jump rope contest.
- Play hopscotch or jacks.
- Plan a menopause potluck with soy recipes.
- Go rollerblading.
- Start an email newsletter sharing funny stories about flashing.
- Plan a weekend getaway.
- Learn new skills or how to begin an investment club.
- Take golf lessons.
- Attend a WNBA game.
- Start a storytelling club.
- Write a cookbook together with healthy soul food recipes.
- Take a kickboxing class.
- Do something unexpected. Take a day off work and meet for tea.
- Take all your old clothes and donate them to a women's shelter.
- Volunteer for a women's group.
- Plan a party and play music from the '70s.
- Celebrate everyone's fiftieth birthday.

Select Some of the Following Topics to Explore and Discuss in Your Group

Affirm your creativity. Maybe you have set priorities in your life that do not leave time for creative pursuits. Did you ever want to paint, draw, dance, or create sculptures? Now is the time to do things we have put off.

Commit to harmony and wholeness in your life. Get your life in order. Eliminate the negative relationships and circumstances that cause you pain. Focus on peace of mind and projects that reflect your values.

Recognize the beauty of your body as it is right now. We all have our own style and beauty. Accentuate the things about your body that please you. Take care of your body and keep it fit. Come to grips with a realistic body image.

Take charge of your midlife journey. This will mean different things for different women. Decide on the way you want your journey to unfold and make it happen.

Celebrate your wisdom and maturity. We have paid our dues and learned from our mistakes. Give yourself credit for what you have achieved.

Educate yourself about African traditions and customs to sustain and affirm your cultural identity.

Follow your own path and do what makes you happy. This involves rejecting the negative expectations of others. This is not our mama's menopause. We have charted a new path and we must do it our way. Use your life energy to be the best. Give yourself permission to let go of old negative experiences that may be limiting you or holding you back

Share your story with other women who will empathize and nurture you.

Let others inspire you with their strategies for success. Discuss your dilemmas. Two heads are better than one.

Explore beliefs about our changing roles and reassure each other that we can overcome all our personal challenges. Sharing our stories helps us learn how to reconcile our inner voice with what we have been conditioned to believe.

Revel in your sexuality and take pleasure in your sexuality regardless of whether or not you have a partner. Trust your inner guide.

Build credibility by keeping your promises to yourself. Whenever we make a promise to others, we try hard to keep our word. In the Second

Half of Life, spend more time and effort honoring the promises you make to yourself.

Don't be afraid to rock the boat.

Do something different in your life. Your choices in the past may have been based on what's best for everyone else. What do you need to do to improve your life now? Evaluate what you need to bring about change in your life. Make new choices. Allow your brilliance to shine through even when it makes others uncomfortable.

Do whatever it takes to get your emotional, spiritual, sexual, and creative needs met. It is often hard for us to ask for what we need or to be honest enough with ourselves to admit our needs. We should be assertive about taking care of our spirits as well as our bodies.

Give your love to someone who loves you and treats you with respect. Express your feelings clearly. Be heard.

Release your anger. Be honest with yourself. Look at the truths you have been avoiding. Take responsibility for your happiness. Take advantage of the lessons learned throughout your menopause journey.

Become a lifelong learner.

Life Lesson

At this stage of my life, I find that taking time to pamper myself is vital to my existence. I take one day per month as my self-care time. Many African-American women everywhere are setting aside more time for themselves. We agree that it is easier to do this as we get older and wiser. It's like we finally recognize the value of pampering ourselves. Ten minutes a day reflecting on your life and being mindful of what's going on in every aspect of your being makes a difference. Relaxing and rejuvenating should become a higher priority. We owe it to ourselves. We need it and we deserve it!

What's It All About in Menopause?

Our physical, mental, and emotional symptoms at menopause may well be part of our initiation process into a wiser, more fulfilling stage of life.

Menopause is about attunement, synchronicity, feeling wonderful, and snatching joy from each day. Develop a greater sense of control during a time when control is hard to come by. Menopause is about "exhaling."

> **"As women go through the pause they seem to arrive at a new place in their lives. They take themselves more seriously. They make major changes in their lives."**
> —*Lonnie Barbach, Ph.D.,*
>   **The Pause**

It doesn't matter if your goal-setting sessions are formal, as long as each person clearly states what she wants to achieve and progress is monitored. Sisters describe a new sense of clarity at midlife about what's important to them. They have been surprised by how much energy they found to achieve their new goals.

Goal Setting

Group meetings provide the perfect opportunity to begin setting goals. The support and guidance of our "sister network" helps us stretch ourselves and dare to talk about the dreams we may have deferred. Goal setting is a skill and there are specific rules to follow that help you set goals properly.

Rule # 1: Strive for balance by setting goals in all the different areas of your life.

Rule #2: Design goals based on your priorities in life. Ask yourself what is of value to you today.

Rule #3: Goals should be in tune. Don't set goals in one area of your life that will conflict with your success in another area.

Rule #4: All goals must be realistic. Set your goals only as far out as you can realistically see. Once you get closer to achieving them, you can reset them.

Rule #5: Make your goals specific and clear. Focus on the details of what you want.

Rule #6: Visualize the final results. Become end result oriented. We are magnetically drawn to the pictures in our minds.

Rule #7: Accountability—you are accountable for the results. We are in charge of our lives and it is up to us to decide what's good enough for us. When we expect more of ourselves, we will achieve more.

MENOPAUSE CALL TO ACTION

♦ Celebrate this passage with other women.
♦ Commit your time and energy to collaborating on enjoying the moment while inventing a better future.
♦ Develop an Afrocentric ritual to add meaning to your Do Menopause with An Attitude meetings.
♦ Plan a yearly retreat.
♦ Select several menopause role models to inspire you to do menopause with heart and soul.
♦ Focus on bringing harmony and balance to your life.

> **"Deal with yourself as an individual worthy of respect and make everyone else deal with you the same way."**
>
> —*Nikki Giovanni*

♦ Set new and exciting midlife goals and use your "sister network" to help you brainstorm and visualize your success.
♦ Express your feelings of fear, vulnerability, or self-doubt so you are authentic in your relationships with these women.
♦ Share your successes and failures.

♦ Proclaim your right to live life with gusto.
♦ Know the value of your legacy to the world.
♦ Invest yourself in a cause that excites you and one that relates to
  midlife goals.
♦ Celebrate! Celebrate! Celebrate!

CHAPTER 11

Become a Leader In Your Life

Menopause is an opportunity for us to embrace change, become leaders in our lives, and set the stage for living our dreams. There are several lessons to learn, including how to cope with change, solve problems, and face our fears. We must engage in the process of looking within to assess our realities and to plan for our futures. According to the theories of psychologist Leon Festinger, there is a great deal of discomfort, or "dissonance," involved in any change. Sometimes people avoid making changes in their lives not because they don't have the ability to change, but because they want to avoid feeling uncomfortable. Girlfriends, it's like our grandmothers used to say, "No pain, no gain." Feeling some discomfort does not have to keep us from achieving positive growth. It may be part of the process, a necessary watershed to future growth.

When I ask sisters about change, they invariably answer that change is a constant in their lives. Sometimes they handle it and sometimes it handles them. Whatever the case, they say they just keep on trucking. I know you know what they're talking about, but let's do more than that. Hearing that old saying about trucking hurts because it brings to mind all the hard work Black women are expected to do without taking the time to follow their bliss and fulfill their dreams. We deserve the joy of creating a lifestyle that nourishes our spirit. We can use this transitional time of life to depend on ourselves, and use our brilliance to make exciting and rewarding things happen in our lives. Let's dig deep and bring to the surface our true essence. Changing our thinking, reframing the issues in our lives, and expressing our feelings are all part of using our minds to help our bodies heal.

Several years ago I developed a program called Survival Skills for Success, which teaches young adults and teens how to enhance their lifestyle management skills. I talk with them about the consequences of their behavior and I try to help them understand how decisions made today will impact their future. A consequence is a direct result of an action or situation. I believe that learning to face consequences builds integrity. This is a lesson that we can benefit from during menopause.

I am who I believe myself to be. With practice, I can always change my opinions and beliefs about myself. When I made a decision to start working for myself, I began to gather experience in consulting on a part-time basis. I negotiated an agreement with my boss, the dean at Columbia Graduate School of Business, to allow me to leave my duties as assistant director of student affairs two days a week at noon to work as a stress management consultant. My rationale was that I couldn't take advantage of the liberal tuition benefits because I had already completed all the required coursework for my doctorate. Allowing me to adjust my work schedule served as a way to compensate me and keep me from leaving my job. They had created this position for me and wanted to keep me, so I had some leverage.

I marketed stress-management seminars to major corporations and led stress-management groups for career women in the evenings. I rented space from a group of women psychologists on 72nd Street and West End Avenue in New York. They offered me phone and mail privileges and the use of beautiful office space for $20 per hour. I was able to start consulting with a very small investment. I made things happen for myself and I still do that. Success hasn't always been easy, but I have developed the ability to be resilient, a good quality for us to have throughout our menopausal journey. I bounce back from my disappointments with a stronger drive to find my way. However, I couldn't have been creative and assertive about my career since reaching menopause without facing my problems with depression, my sexuality, and dealing with my menopausal symptoms effectively.

I developed my own training materials and consulted with agencies that provided services for female substance abusers and runaway teens. All of these experiences prepared me for running my own education and training corporation, which is what I do today. I took a risk and it paid off. My colleagues tried to discourage me because the professors at Columbia Business School were encouraged to have consulting contracts, but not the officers. All I had to do was challenge the status quo. I asserted myself and reminded the dean of my marketable skills. He didn't know I had no clue of how to be a consultant. After he approved my schedule, I took the leap and became one.

In order to be truly happy in life, I had to create the kind of working situation that suited me. In the process of making this happen, I boosted my self-esteem, expanded my comfort zones, and controlled my self-talk. These are the types of thinking strategies that are most important if we are ever going to start living for ourselves and making sure that we are doing the kind of work that validates who we are. Sometimes I meet women who are very creative but feel stifled by their jobs. It's hard for them to use all of their potential because each day is a chore. They feel that life is passing them by. In spite of the fact that they feel boxed in by all their responsibilities, I teach them to focus on creative ways to make changes. What can you learn from your past experiences? How can you use the memory of those experiences to help you today?

Celebrating the Second Half of Life can only bring about positive consequences. Since we are going to go through this passage, we might as well set goals to change by intent. Refusing to plan and design your own approach means that you will be unprepared and have even less control over your passage. I am sure you, like me, prefer to do things by intent and to prepare yourself mentally and physically for each new step.

THERE ARE CERTAIN FACTS ABOUT CHANGE WE NEED TO THINK ABOUT:

♦ Although change is inevitable, how we cope with it is up to us.
♦ People who have high self-esteem feel a sense of inner security that lets them know they are capable of handling change.
♦ Resilient people master change because they know how to bounce back from disappointment or defeat. They keep moving forward and taking risks even when they can't predict outcomes.
♦ Resisting change is pointless.
♦ Mastering change keeps us from being a victim of change.

I have encouraged you to anticipate how your body will change and then figure out what you want to do to cope with these changes. What do you say to yourself when you are facing a challenge or feeling overwhelmed by the changes in your environment? Use your inner resources to adjust. You may need to develop new coping skills, thinking skills, and a higher level of self-awareness. Think about it. Can you build and maintain high self-esteem when the world is bombarding you with so many negative images of African-American women? Does the fact that we are expected to conform to the "almost white" standards of beauty like Halle Barry impact our level of self-esteem at midlife? She won the Oscar for Best Actress, but was that a tribute to her considerable talent, or was the message that Black women have to be outstanding and conform to white standards of beauty in order to be recognized? If that is true, how does it make you feel? Are you focusing on the losses or the gains at midlife?

Learn to Cope With Change and Make It Work For You

Times of change often force us to stop and reevaluate the quality of our lives. If you are not happy, menopause is a perfect moment to make your life serve your inner needs. Make a commitment to do what feels good. In our business, we often get the opportunity to work with dislocated managers and executives. Many customers call us after completing the grieving process to tell us they have started their own business or found more meaningful careers. The painful process of losing a job leads to something better. In the Second Half of Life, our struggles to cope with new changes can compel us to design a better future. Managing change is a skill.

What are the major attributes we need to develop in order to master change successfully during perimenopause/menopause?

- Courage
- Resilience
- Focus
- Willingness to change
- Enhanced self-awareness

- Flexibility
- Persistence
- Open mindedness
- Creativity

AFFIRMATIONS
- Developing courage at midlife helps me take risks in my personal and professional life.
- I use my unlimited power to build an exciting and meaningful Second Half of Life.
- I feel vibrantly healthy and effervescently happy every day.

Perimenopause kind of slipped by me with minimal awareness, but I chose to handle menopause in a creative way by focusing on the opportunity to learn new skills and increase my level of self-awareness. I made a decision to learn as much as I could about the transition, and I gained in other ways. The research involved led me to spend time online visiting women's health websites and increasing my proficiency in browsing cyberspace. It helped me prepare to write this book and also helped me locate my online Ph.D. program in natural health.

There are times when a significant emotional event causes us to decide to change. When my second stepfather, who was the kindest man I ever met, died a painful death from cancer in 1991, it was a major turning point in my life. I found myself eliminating the things in my life that were stressful and trivial. I grew a great deal in a short period of time and felt as though I was in the "zone." I am going through a similar, but more powerful, type of metamorphosis at menopause. I am very conscious of needing to prepare myself for change. Actually, I was hurled into making changes in my perceptions about almost every aspect of my life. You can make the same commitment to planning for your future.

Plan For Change

Change is often quite unpredictable even when we attempt to prepare for it and anticipate what will be required of us. We have to deal with changes related to our shifting roles with family members and differences in what is expected at work in combination with all the biological changes. It is a mix unlike anything we have ever experienced. Although we have a great deal of experience in handling a multitude of tasks, we shouldn't assume our old strategies will be effective in this new phase of our lives.

Mastering these changes requires us to develop new ways of behaving and new thinking skills. All lasting change starts from within. African-American women have been successfully completing the task of changing and reinventing themselves for centuries. Adjusting and adapting to change is a lifelong task and we do it well. The key is to be more conscious of changing effectively in a manner consistent with our goals.

Jon R. Katzenbach, author of *Real Change Leaders*, describes change leaders as people who are able to bring about change in organizations by mobilizing others to increase performance and exceed organizational goals. He states, "Real Change Leaders do not care if the change effort is fast or slow, empowered or controlled, one-time, recurring, cultural or engineered—or all of the above. They only care that it is people intensive, and performance oriented."

This concept is relevant to us in our personal lives. No matter where we are on the change pendulum, once we enter midlife we need to empower ourselves to increase our performance. I see us mobilizing ourselves to use all of our potential. Once we are past the turbulence or what Dr. Levy calls "flux," we can begin to develop positive energy to take us where we choose to be.

They are many ways for us to plan for change and the first step involves understanding why change is necessary.

TIPS ON MANAGING CHANGE

It's hard to change without feeling a sense of urgency. We feel complacent. You might be saying, "Why change when everything seems great the way it is?" But change by nature requires some movement and there's always room for improvement. We have no choice about the physical changes taking place in our bodies, but we are in control of how we respond psychologically, spiritually, and emotionally.

Transformations take place when you push yourself. I'm not talking about being "superwomen." We've been there, done that and bought the T-shirt, or maybe in our case bought the whole designer outfit. I'm talking about saying, "I am totally committed to making big-time changes in the way that I talk to myself, the way I allow other people to treat me, and the way I take advantage of opportunities. I tell myself menopause is my time to shine." Transformation becomes possible when we eliminate the barriers to success, those self-imposed mental and emotional obstacles that hold us back. It could be fear of the unknown or fear of success. We need to expand our comfort zone, as Dr. Susan Jeffers writes in *Feel the Fear and Do It Anyway:* "Fears reflect your sense of self and your ability to handle this world." She encourages people to face theirs by taking action right away. Don't wait until you are no longer afraid before taking the first step in a new direction.

Sometimes we avoid change because we're in denial about the need for change, or because we're so busy with all of the other "stuff" in our lives. Dealing with change effectively takes hard work and serious thought. You probably feel like you already have enough to think about. I know I felt like I didn't have time for menopause, but like they say, time waits for no one.

Insist on a higher level of honesty with yourself. Take an objective, hard look at yourself and evaluate what's going on in every area of your life. Face the current reality of your existence and then make a true commitment to changing every single thing that bothers you. Once you take a hard look at where you are, you can begin to set goals for a new future. Spend as much time as possible working on getting what you want. Always focus on and think about what you want. Check yourself on your level of life satisfaction. Are you satisfied with your personal life and spiritual life, relationships, educational goals, career goals, and your level of mental health and physical health?

Here is an example of how one change can lead to another and you can invent your future based on new goals or revisiting old forgotten goals. I've been traveling thousands of miles each year working with all types of organizations and with people from all walks of life. But my true passion has always been helping women. Prior to menopause, I spent several years forgetting how much I enjoy teaching and learning from other women. Following my heart, evaluating my life, and meeting women who are living their dreams

> **"The greatest rewards come only from the greatest commitment."**
> —*Arlene Blum*

motivated me to start making plans to do what I really want to do. You can't predict the people or the circumstances that will inspire you. Are you successful at inspiring yourself? What does it take to get you excited about your future?

Life Lesson

Menopause can be a peak experience. The famous psychologist Abraham Maslow describes a peak experience as a moment of bliss or incredible joy. People who report having this type of experience describe these moments as pure, positive happiness when all doubts, all fears, all inhibitions, all tensions, and all weaknesses, were left behind.

After this experience, people tend to feel great insight, creativity, or inspiration that takes them on a journey to a new place in their world. "Menopause

Moments" can be like a peak experience. There are moments when you feel in tune, centered, grounded, and spiritually intact. You know how powerful and gifted you are in every aspect of your being.

Sharon, a forty-eight-year-old successful lawyer, took risks during menopause and changed careers. When she started menopause, she admitted to herself that she was unhappy with her career and felt the need to do something more creative. She decided to take pottery classes in her spare time at her local community center. Soon she found herself spending every spare moment creating wonderful gifts for her friends and family. She put her bowls and vases on consignment in several gift shops and quickly found that she had more orders than she could handle. Her hobby became a full-time business. Today she has four employees, her own shop, and a thriving Web-based business. She's happier than she has ever been. She enthusiastically looks forward to each new day. She explains, "I couldn't face corporate life another day even though I loved the money and prestige. It wasn't me anymore. I needed to express myself differently. I wanted my next thirty years to be more fulfilling."

> **"I always had only one prayer: Lord, just crack the door a little bit, and I'll kick it open all the way."**
> —*Shirley Caesar*

At this time in our lives, we need to become leaders in our own personal lifestyle. We may already be leaders in our careers and in our professional lives, but we may not be cognizant of applying the same degree of creativity, innovativeness, and renewal in our personal lives.

LEADERSHIP

John P. Kotter, author of *Leading Change*, defines leadership as follows: "Leadership defines what the future should look like, aligns people with that vision, and inspires them to make it happen despite the obstacles."

Leaders turn challenges into opportunities. The challenge of mastering menopause

> "The path from dependence to independence teaches us about rejection, discomfort, and pain."
> —*Chip R. Bell,* Managers as Mentors

is also an opportunity to make our lives better. Sisters, I'm talking about reengineering our lives so that all of our needs are being met. Ask yourself the question, "What's good enough for me?" Maybe being satisfied isn't enough. How about designing your Second Half of Life so that it greatly exceeds your expectations?

Leaders take risks and never settle. Improve your standards of excellence during midlife and then use your strengths in planning, organizing, and goal setting to make things happen for you. What have you planned to do in the next ten years? How are these plans different from the plans you made at age thirty-five? The period between age forty-five and fifty-five is a pivotal phase.

Good leaders envision success. It is imperative for us to have a clear picture of the way we want our lives to be. Remember, our minds are so strong, remarkable, and powerful that once we envision something with emotion, our reticular activating system, a netlike group of cells at the base of the brain that acts as a filter for information and sensory messages, allows information to get through to help us move toward our goals.

What is your vision for life after menopause? The choices, attitudes, and expectations that you have today will shape your future. If you love the life you have now and everything is perfect, then you can refuse to grow. But if you are like most of us, there's always room for improvement. Make life what you want it to be. Use the gifts of your mind and brain to help you do this. Clear visions give us a track to follow. They help us focus on where we're going. They give us benchmarks for measuring our progress.

Develop a new "mental model" of life after menopause. In *The Fifth Discipline*, Peter Senge talks about how "mental models" are composed of our expectations and beliefs that influence the way we see our world and the way we behave when we are faced with change in our lives. Once we alter our perception of menopause, we will view our Second Half of Life from a different point of view. He describes personal mastery as a high level of achievement or skill development in a particular area of learning. Our enjoyment of our lives at midlife will increase once we improve our personal mastery of the challenges of this transition. What is your "mental model" of menopause? How would you rate your level of personal mastery of midlife transition?

Build a higher level of positive regard. Psychologist Carl Rogers taught us that unconditional positive regard is the most important factor in developing positive self-esteem and self-confidence. Accepting yourself and your feelings about who you are, regardless of the mistakes you have made in the past, helps to build positive regard. Become your own best girlfriend. Think about your strengths. How has your level of positive self-regard helped you achieve your goals in the past? We can use more personal power and self-love at this turning point in our lives.

Develop a positive expectancy for the future. Look forward to a happier, abundant, and fulfilling Second Half of Life. We need to give ourselves permission to have the best life has to offer, with a focus on what's good for us. Let's let our loved ones learn how to fight some of their own battles. The universal law of attraction states we will only attract to ourselves those things we honestly feel we deserve. If you want something better, you will create if for yourself. What do you believe is good enough for you?

Understand that optimism is an attitude. As stated in *The Power of Optimism* by Alan Loy McGinnis, "Optimists are challenged by their problems. They develop mental techniques and habits of thought that help them excel." He found that some of the most optimistic people had very unhappy childhoods, so they had a lot of practice in learning how to focus on the positive. Optimism will help us do menopause with a new attitude.

> **"When we begin to love and approve of ourselves, it's amazing how our lives change."**
> —*Louise Hay*

Develop effective thinking about menopause. The word "thinking" means to ponder, contemplate, study, reflect, use logic, and deliberate, according to *Webster's Collegiate Dictionary*. Effective thinking takes us to a reasonable conclusion where we make better decisions. The quality of our decisions during menopause will be based on the quality of our thinking.

ENHANCE YOUR PROBLEM-SOLVING SKILLS AT MIDLIFE

Problem solving involves finding answers, seeking solutions, and resolving problems.

The steps to solving problems are:

1. State the problem.
2. Clearly define the problem.
3. Brainstorm action steps.
4. Develop a plan.
5. Put it into action.
6. Evaluate the success of the plan.
7. Determine if the plan can be improved.
8. Fine-tune and adjust the plan.

What midlife issues and problems do you want to address? Try the following on for size.

- Improve your self-image and self-esteem by accepting your body the way it is, or solve the problem by taking action to lose weight, firm up, build muscle, or whatever it takes.
- Eliminate negative thoughts about yourself. Resolve your esteem issues. Understand the true meaning of self-esteem. Women with high self-esteem are much more likely to take care of themselves and achieve optimal physical and mental health. Once we develop sufficient self-esteem, we will be less influenced by negative thoughts and events.
- Use menopause as an opportunity to learn how to accept yourself with all your idiosyncrasies, thought patterns, and weaknesses.
- Celebrate menopause by solving your problems from a new perspective so that you can achieve more of your goals after menopause.

Good problem solving also involves developing cognitive strategies that help you think critically and formulate problems accurately. After successfully solving problems, it is easy for us to make wise decisions about the next thirty years of our lives. Ian Mitroff, in *Smart Thinking for Crazy Times,* urges us to question our assumptions before starting to solve our problems. Figure out what you need to help you solve problems. Perhaps you need more information, specific skills, or someone to listen to you.

As you define your problems at midlife, stop worrying about them, and take action, you will begin solving them with brilliance. "Worry is the thinking part of anxiety. Intense worry is about as useful to our thinking as lighted matches in a dynamite factory." This is how H. Norman Wright discusses the nature of worrying in *Winning Over Your Emotions.*

I define worrying as negative goal-setting because it focuses our energy on the problems without focusing on the solutions. Start seeing solutions in your mind immediately after defining each problem. Rehearse several possible outcomes and see how they fit. Tell yourself the solutions to all your problems exist; you just don't see them yet. Put your problems in per-spective by asking yourself if anyone has ever experienced this type of problem before.

USE YOUR INTUITION

Our hunches are based on innate wisdom that is hard to understand. Taking an intu-itive approach to the Second Half of Life will help us get in touch with our feelings.

> "We have all heard of women's intuition, but not all of us use it to empower ourselves."
> —*Beth Moran,*
> **Intuitive Healing**

Think about all the times in your life where you didn't pay attention to your hunches and you regretted it later. It's easier to do this when you give yourself permission to take risks because you know you are bigger than the problems that you face.

Doc Talk — Dr. Barbara Levy

Some of us experience this journey as a wonderful trip with smooth, calm seas and warm breezes, but for many of us the waters are fairly stormy…more like a gale or a roller coaster than a pleasant vacation. Menopause is our body saying, "Hello, I'm here." Ask yourself if your body is screaming at you with a wake-up call. Use your women's ways of knowing to help you find the answer. There is no choice but to change, our bodies won't give us any other option. So…we can either suffer with the physical and emotional distress of menopause or we can heed the wake-up call to make the changes necessary to feel our best.

Adopt Habits to a Successful Menopause

♦ Use this chance to change by intent.

♦ Live your life to the fullest right now.

♦ See menopause as a gateway to achieving new heights.

♦ Take risks to make things happen for you.

♦ Blaze your own trails.

♦ Open yourself to new horizons.

♦ Be part of a cause bigger than yourself; do things for the greater good.

♦ Surround yourself with people who inspire you and support you.

♦ Design your own legacy and take a stand for what you believe.

♦ Have some fun every day. One day a week, try to have too much fun.

♦ Be proud of who you are at every stage of your life. People notice *when and where we enter.*

♦ Find out what makes you happy, then do it.

♦ See menopause as a journey to renewal.

♦ When things seem impossible, do them anyway. Remember, *we specialize in the wholly impossible.*

♦ Proclaim your Second Half of Life as your time to be free of any limitations or losses.

Menopause Call To Action

In the Second Half of Life, make a commitment to take charge of your mental, spiritual, and physical health.

♦ Boost your self-esteem so that you put your health first.

♦ Learn about the healing power of your body.

♦ Concentrate on strategies that take into account the mind and body connection.

♦ Focus on wellness practices that correct imbalances in your body and decrease your exposure to toxins.

- Make use of complementary medicine to manage nutrition, exercise, chronic conditions, and symptoms.
- Seek out medical doctors who value holistic health care and are willing to work with you with a combination of traditional allopathic medicine as well as natural remedies.
- Shake things up. Shift those gears.
- Love what you do or find something else to do. Life is too short to go through the motions of living everyday.
- Focus on your strengths, your passion, and the courage that is our legacy from the strong and wise African-American women who have come before us.

Suggested Reading

Anderson, Bob. *Stretching*. Bolinas, CA: Shelter Publications, 1980.

Anderson, Jean. *Sin-Free Desserts*. New York: Doubleday, 1991.

Andrews, Lynn V., and Joyner, Ginny. *Woman at the Edge of Two Worlds.* New York: HarperCollins, 1994.

Barbach, Lonnie, Ph.D. *The Pause: Positive Approaches to Perimenopause & Menopause.* New York: Dutton/Plume, 2002.

Barry, Frank, M.D., and Swinney, Bridget. *The Healthy Heart Formula.* New York: John Wiley & Sons, 1996.

Borysenko, Joan. *Fire in the Soul: A New Psychology of A spiritual Optimism.* New York: Warner Books, 1993.

Boyd, Julia. *Can I Get A Witness: Black Women & Depression.* New York: Dutton/Plume, 1999.

Bricklin, Mark. *Prevention's Practical Encyclopedia of Walking for Health.* Emmaus, PA: Rodale Press, 1992.

Budoff, Penny Wise. *No More Hot Flashes...and Even More Good News.* New York: Warner Books, 1999.

Cabot, Sandra. *Smart Medicine for Menopause: Hormone Replacement Therapy and Its Natural Alternatives.* Garden City Park, NY: Avery Publishing, 1995.

Chopra, Deepak. *The Seven Spiritual Laws of Success: A Practical Guide to the Fulfillment of Your Dreams.* Farmington Hills, MI: Macmillan, 2001.

Cobb, Janine O. *Understanding Menopause: Answers and Advice for Women in the Prime of Life.* New York: Dutton/Plume, 1993.

Cone, Faye K. *Making Sense of Menopause: Over 150 Women and Experts Share Their Wisdom, Experience, and Commonsense Advice.* New York: Simon & Schuster, 1993.

Danquah, Meri Nana-Ama. *Willow Weep For Me: A Black Woman's Journey through Depression.* New York: Ballantine Publishing, 1999.

Dossey, Larry. *Healing Words: The Power of Prayer and the Practice of Medicine.* San Francisco: HarperCollins, 1995.

Finn, Susan. *The Real Life Nutrition Book.* New York: Penguin Books, 1992.

Frances, Allen, M.D., and First, Michael B., M.D. *Your Mental Health: A Layman's Guide to the Psychiatrist's Bible.* New York: Simon & Schuster, 1999.

Gillespie, Clark M.D. *Hormones, Hot Flashes, and Mood Swings: Living Through the Ups and Downs of Menopause.* New York: HarperTrade, 1989.

Gittleman, Ann Louise. *Super Nutrition for Menopause: Take Control of Your Life and Enjoy New Vitality.* Garden City Park, NY: Avery Publishing, 1998.

Gittleman, Ann Louise, and Wright, Jonathan V. *Before the Change: Taking Charge of Your Perimenopause.* San Francisco: HarperCollins Publishers, 1999.

Goldstein, Steven R. *Could It Be Perimenopause?* New York: Little, Brown & Company, 2000.

Greenwood, Sadja, and Quackenbush, Marcia. *Menopause, Naturally: Preparing for the Second Half of Life.* New York: Volcan Press, 1996.

Greer, Germaine. *The Change: Women, Aging and the Menopause.* New York: Fawcett, 1993.

Grundy, Scott. (Ed.) *Low-Fat, Low Cholesterol Cookbook*. New York: Random House, 1989.

Guy-Sheftall, Beverly. *Words of Fire: An Anthology of African American Feminist Thought*. New York: New Press, 1995.

Hay, Louise. *The Power Is Within You.* Carson, CA: Hay House, 1991.

Heber, David, MD. *Natural Remedies for a Healthy Heart*. Garden City Park, NY: Avery Publishing, 1998.

Hammer, Michael. "Reengineering Work: Don't Automate, Obliterate." *Harvard Business Review*, July-August 1990, 104-11.

Hiser, Elizabeth. *The Other Diabetes: Living and Eating Well with Type 2 Diabetes*. New York: Morrow, 1999.

Hogan, R., Gordon C., & Hogan, J. "What We Know About Leadership." *American Psychologist*, June 1994, 493-504.

Jacobowitz, Ruth S. *150 Most-Asked Questions About Menopause: What Women Really Want to Know*. New York: HarperCollins, 1996.

Jacobowitz, Ruth S. *Estrogen Answer Book*. New York: Little, Brown & Company, 1999.

Jacobs, Harriet A. *Incidents In the Life of a Slave Girl*. Cambridge, MA: Harvard University Press, 1987.

Jeffers, Susan Ph.D. *End the Struggle and Dance with Life: How to Build Yourself Up When the World Gets You Down.* Collingdale, PA: DIANE Publishing, 1998.

Jeffers, Susan Ph.D. *Feel the Fear and Do It Anyway: Dynamic Techniques for Turning Fear, Indecision, and Anger into Power, Action, and Love*. New York: Fawcett, 1996.

Jeffers, Susan. Ph.D. *Opening Our Hearts to Men*. New York: Fawcett, 1990.

Kabat-Zinn, Jon. *Mindfulness Meditation in Everyday Life*. New York: Hyperion, 1994.

Kushner, Harold. *When All You've Ever Wanted Isn't Enough*. New York: Summet Books, 1986.

Lark, Susan M. *The Estrogen Decision: Self Help Book*. Berkeley, CA: Celestial Arts Publishing, 1996.

Lawrence, Marcia. *Menopause and Madness: The Truth About Estrogen and the Mind*. Bridgewater, NJ: Replica Books, 2000.

Lee, John R., and Hopkins, Virginia L. *What Your Doctor May Not Tell You About Menopause: The Breakthrough Book on Natural Progesterone*. New York: Warner Books, 2001.

Mayo, Mary Ann, and Mayo, Joseph L. *The Menopause Manager: A Safe Path for a Natural Change*. Ada, MI: Fleming H. Revell, 2000.

Morton, Patricia. *Disfigured Images: The Historical Assault on Afro-American Women*. Westport, CT: Greenwood Publishing, 1991.

Moquette-Magee, Elaine. *Eat Well for a Healthy Menopause: The Low-Fat, High-Nutrition Guide*. New York: John Wiley & Sons, 1996.

Ojeda, Linda Ph.D. *Menopause Without Medicine: Feel Healthy, Look Younger, Live Longer*. Alameda, CA: Hunter House, 2000.

Perry, Susan. *Natural Menopause: The Complete Guide*. New York: Perseus Books Group, 2000.

Rako, Susan M.D. *The Hormone of Desire: The Truth About Testosterone, Sexuality, and Menopause*. New York: Harmony Books, 1999.

Roth, Geneen. *When Food Is Love*. New York: Penguin Books, 1991.

Sands, Gayle. *Is It Hot in Here or Is It Me? A Personal Look at the Facts, Fallacies, and Feelings of Menopause*. New York: HarperCollins, 1994.

Schultz, Carol R., and Jenkins, Mary. *60 Second Menopause Management: The Quickest Ways to Handle Problems and Discomforts.* Far Hills, NJ: New Horizon Press Publishers, 1995.

Schlesinger, Sarah. *500 (Practically) Fat-Free One Pot Recipes.* New York: Villard Books/Random House, 1994.

Shandler, Nina. *Estrogen: The Natural Way: Over 250 Easy and Delicious Recipes for Menopause.* Collingdale, PA: DIANE Publishing, 2002.

Smith, Barbara. *Home Girls: A Black Feminist Anthology.* New York: Kitchen Table: Women of Color Press, 1983.

Stillerman, Elaine. *The Encyclopedia of Bodywork: From Acupressure to Zone Therapy.* New York: Facts on File, 1997.

Turkington, Carol, and Johnson, Susan. *The Perimenopause Handbook.* New York: Contemporary Books, 1998.

Wade, Brenda, Ph.D., and Richardson, Brenda Lane. *What Mama Couldn't Tell Us About Love.* Collingdale, PA: DIANE Publishing, 2001.

Warga, Claire L., Ph.D. *Menopause and the Mind: The Complete Guide to Coping with the Cognitive Effects of Perimenopause and Menopause.* New York: Simon & Schuster, 2000.

Waterhouse, Debra. *Outsmarting the Midlife Fat Cell: Winning Weight Control Strategies for Women over 35 to Stay Fit Through Menopause.* New York: Hyperion Press, 1999.

Weed, Susan S. *New Menopausal Years, The Wise Woman Way: Alternative Approaches for Women 30-90.* Saugerties, NY: Ash Tree Publishing, 2000.

Weinstock, Lorna, Gilman, Eleanor. *Overcoming Panic Disorder: A Women's Guide.* New York: Contemporary Books, 1998.

Yates, Beverly, M.D. *Heart Health for Black Women: A Natural Approach to Healing and Preventing Heart Disease.* New York: Avalon Publishing, 2000.

APPENDIX B

Resources

Alliance for Alternatives in Health Care
P.O. Box 5167
West Hills, CA 91308
818-226-9829
FAX: 818-226-9820

American Association of Naturopathic Physicians
3201 New Mexico Avenue, NW
Suite 350
Washington, DC 20016
202-895-1392
TOLL FREE: 866-538-2267
FAX: 202-274-1992
member.services@naturopathic.com

American Foundation of Traditional Chinese Medicine
505 Beach Street
San Francisco, CA 94133
415-392-7002
FAX: 415-392-7003

American Holistic Medical Association
12101 Menaul Blvd NE
Suite C
Albuquerque, NM 87112
505-292-7788
FAX: 505-293-7582

American Massage Therapy Association
820 Davis Street, Suite 100
Evanston, IL 60201
847-864-0123
FAX: 847-864-1178

Image Paths, Inc.
891 Moe Drive, Suite C
Akron, OH 44310
TOLL FREE: 800-800-8661
FAX: 330-633-3778

International Chiropractors Association
1110 North Glebe Road, Suite 1000
Arlington, VA 22201
TOLL FREE: 800-423-4690
FAX: 703-528-5023

International College of Traditional Chinese
Medicine of Vancouver
1508 West Broadway Suite 201
Vancouver, BC Canada V6J 1W8
604-731-2926
www.tcmcollege.com

International Institute of Reflexology
5650 First Avenue North
P.O. Box 12642
St. Petersburg, FL 33733-2642
727-343-4811
FAX: 727-381-2807

National Acupuncture and Oriental Medicine Alliance
14637 Starr Road, SE
Olalla, WA 98359
253-851-6896
FAX: 253-851-6833

National Center for Homeopathy
801 North Fairfax Street, Suite 306
Alexandria, VA 22314
TOLL FREE: 877-624-0613
FAX: 708-548-7792

National College of Naturopathic Medicine
049 SW Porter St.
Portland, OR 97201
503-499-4343
FAX: 503-499-0027

National Osteoporosis Foundation
2100 M Street NW
Washington, D.C. 20037-1292
202-223-2226

Reflexology Research
P.O. Box 35820
Albuquerque, NM 87176-5820
505-344-9392
FAX: 505-344-0246

APPENDIX C

Newsletters

A Friend Indeed
P.O. Box 260
Pembina, ND 58271-0260
204-989-8028

Hot Flash
The National Action Forum for Midlife & Older Women
P.O. Box 816
Stony Brook, NY 11790-0609

Menopause News
2074 Union Street
San Francisco, CA 94123

Menopause Today
Planned Parenthood Federation of America
434 W. 33 St.
New York, NY 10001
212-541-7800
FAX: 212-245-1845

National Women's Health Network
514 Tenth Street NW #400
Washington, D.C. 20004
202-628-7814 (voice orders only)
202-347-1140
FAX: 202-347-1168

The Nutrition Action Health Letter
Center for Science in the Public Interest
1875 Connecticut Avenue, NW, Suite 300
Washington, D.C. 20009-5728
202-332-9111

Older Women's League
666 Eleventh Street NW, Suite 700
Washington, D.C. 20001
TOLL FREE: 800-825-3695
202-783-6686
FAX: 202-638-2356

APPENDIX D

Organizations

American College of Cardiology
Heart House
9111 Old Georgetown Road
Bethesda, MD 20814-1699
TOLL FREE: (800) 253-4636 ext. 694
(301) 897-5400
FAX: (301) 897-9745

American College of Women's Health Physicians
1111 N. Plaza Drive, Ste. 550
Schaumburg, IL 60173
(847) 517-7402
FAX: (847) 517-7229

American Diabetes Association
1701 North Beauregard Street
Alexandria, VA 22311
TOLL FREE: (800) 342-2383

American Heart Association
7272 Greenville Avenue
Dallas, TX 75231
TOLL FREE: (800) 242-8721

American Society for Clinical Nutrition
9650 Rockville Pike
Suite L4500
Bethesda, MD 20814-3990
(301) 530-7050

American Menopause Foundation
National Headquarters
350 Fifth Avenue
Suite 2822
New York, NY 10118
(212) 714-2398

Association of Black Psychologists
P.O. Box 55999
Washington, DC 20040-5999

Black Psychiatrists of America
c/o Ramona Davis, M.D., president
866 Carlston Ave.
Oakland, CA 94610
(510) 834-7103

Black Women's Health Study
Stone Epidemiology Unit
1371 Beacon Street
Brookline, MA 02446-9906
TOLL FREE: (800) 786-0814

The National Association of Black Social Workers
8436 West McNichols Avenue
Detroit, MI 48221
(313) 862-6700

National Black Nurses Association
8630 Fenton Street
Suite 330
Silver Spring, MD 20910-3803
(301) 589-3200

National Black Women's Health Project
600 Pennsylvania Ave., SE
Suite 310
Washington, D.C. 20003
(202) 548-4000
FAX: (202) 543-9743

National Mental Health Association
2001 N. Beauregard St., 12 Floor
Alexandria, VA 22311
(703) 684-7722
FAX: (703) 684-5968

Native American Women's Health Education Resource Center
P.O. Box 572
Lake Andes, SD 57356-0572
(605) 487-7072
EMAIL: nativewomen@igc.apc.org

North American Menopause Society (NAMS)
P.O. Box 94527
Cleveland, OH 44101-4527
(440) 442-7550
FAX: (440)442-2660
www.menopause.org

Real Women Project
P.O. Box 90669
San Diego, CA 92169

APPENDIX E

Online Resources

---

www.nami.org
National Alliance for the Mentally Ill

www.healthywomen.org
National Women's Health Resource Center

www.4woman.gov
National Women's Health Information Center

www.hsph.harvard.edu/grhf/WoC
Women of Color Web

www.blackwomenshealth.com
Medical information for African-American women

www.menopauseanswers.com
General information on celebrating menopause

www.essence.com
Health, beauty, entertainment, current events, and lifestyle information for African-American women

www.ebony.com
General topics of interest and current medical information for African-Americans

www.healthjourneys.com
Guided imagery products and wellness information

Notes

Chapter 1

Dyer, Dwayne. *Manifest Your Destiny: The Nine Spiritual Principles for Getting Everything You Want.* New York: HarperCollins, 1997: 78.

Carlson, Richard. *Don't Sweat the Small Stuff Workbook.* New York: Hyperion, 1998.

Bandura, Albert. *Social Foundations of Thought and Action, A Social Cognitive Theory.* Englewood Cliffs, NJ: Prentice Hall, 1986: 1-22.

McGinnis, Alan Loy. *The Power of Optimism.* New York: Harper & Row, 1990.

Chapter 2

Jean-Murat, Carolle, M.D. *Menopause Made Easy.* Carlsbad, CA: Hay House, Inc., 1999: 216.

Romoff, Adam, M.D. with Ina Yalof. *Estrogen, How and Why It Can Save Your Life.* New York: Golden Books, 1999: 33-35.

Kessenich, Linda. "Osteoporosis and African-American Women." *Women's Health Issues,* Vol. 10, No. 6, Nov/Dec 2000.

Weaver, Roniece, ct al. *Slim Down Sister: African American Women's Guide to Healthy, Permanent Weight Loss*. New York, NY: Plume, 2001: 1-7.

Chapter 3

Selye, Hans. *The Stress of Life*. New York: McGraw-Hill, 1978.

Chapter 4

Landau, Carol, Ph.D., Cyr, Michele G, M.D. and Anne W. Moulton, M.D. *The Complete Book of Menopause*. New York: Berkley Publishing Group, 1994.

Steege, John F., M.D., Metzer, Deborah A., Ph.D., M.D. and Barbara S. Levy, M.D. *Chronic Pelvic Pain: An Integrated Approach*. Philadelphia: W.B. Saunders Company, 1997.

Schwartz, Alan N., M.D., Jimenez, Richard, M.D., Myers, Tracy, M.H.A. and Andrew Solomon, M.D. *Getting The Best From Your Doctor*. Minneapolis, MN: Chronomed Publishing, 1998: 6-7.

Chapter 5

Skog, Susan. *Depression: What Your Body's Trying to Tell You*. New York: Hearst Books, 1999: 3.

Zuess, Johnathan, M.D. *The Wisdom of Depression*. New York: Harmony Books, 1998.

Schultz, Mona Lisa. *Awakening Intuition: Using Your Mind-Body Network for Insight and Healing*. New York: Harmony Books, 1998.

Bloodworth, Veniece. *Key to Yourself*. Marina Del Ray, CA: DeVorss & Co., 1980.

Davis, Laura, and Ellen Bass. *The Courage to Heal*. New York: Harper & Row, 1992: 58-59.

Brandon, Nathaniel, Ph.D. *The Power of Self-Esteem*. New York: AMACOM, a division of the American Management Association, 1994.

Romoff, Adam, M.D. with Inca Yalof. *Estrogen: How and Why It Can Save Your Life*. New York: Golden Books, 1999.

Ford, Gilliam. *Listening to Your Hormones*. Rocklin, CA: Prima Publishing, 1996, 55.

Wade, Brenda, Ph.D. and Brenda Lane Richardson. *What Mama Couldn't Tell Us About Love*. New York: Harper Collins Books, 1999: xix, 29.

Chapter 6

hooks, bell. *Sisters of the Yam: Black Women and Self-Recovery*. Boston: South End Press, 1993.

Mitchell, Angela with Kennise Herring, Ph.D. *What the Blues Is All About*. New York: Berkley Publishing Group, 1998, 156.

Goldsby Grant, Gwendolyn. *The Best Kind of Loving: A Black Woman's Guide to Finding Intimacy*. New York: Harper Perennial, 1995, 10-11.

Chapter 7

Rako, Susan M.D. *The Hormone of Desire*. New York: Three Rivers Press, 1996: 54.

Morgan, Joan. *When Chickenheads Come Home to Roost*. New York: Touchstone Books, 1999.

Chapter 8

Yates, Beverly, M.D. *Heart Health for Black Women.* New York: Marlowe & Company, 2000: 42-43.

Walker, Marcellus, A, M.D. and Kenneth B. Singleton, M.D. *Natural Health for African Americans.* New York, NY: Warner Books, 1999.

Nelson, Miriam, Ph.D. and Sarah Wernick, Ph.D. *Strong Women Stay Young.* New York: Bantam Books, 1997: 7-13.

Hammond, Christopher. *Homeopathy.* New York: Time Life Books, 1995: 11.

Clark Hine, Darlene. *Black Women in America.* New York: Facts on File Books, 1997: 119-120.

Gittleman, Louise. *Supernutrition for Menopause.* Garden City, NY: Avery Publishing Group, 1998: 6.

Kushi, Michio. *The Macrobiotic Way.* Garden City, NY: Avery Books, 1993: 59-82.

Chapter 9

Lu, Henry C., Ph.D. *Chinese Natural Cures.* New York: Black Dog & Leventhal Publishers, Inc., 1994: 10-14, 302-308.

Reese, Sara Lomax, editor, Johnson, Kirk and Therman Evans, M.D. *Staying Strong.* New York: Avon books, 1999: 3-43.

Townes, Emilie, M. *Breaking the Fine Rain of Death.* New York: Continum, 63.

Micco Snow, Alice and Susan Enns Stans. *Healing Plants.* Gainesville, FL: University Press of Florida, 2001: 38-51.

Ojeda, Linda. *Menopause Without Medicine.* Alameda, CA: Hunter House, Inc., 1995: 37-45.

Chapter 10

Reese, Sara Lomax, editor, Johnson, Kirk and Therman Evans, M.D. *Staying Strong.* New York: Avon books, 1999: 17, 21, 35.

Jones, Laurie Beth. *The Path.* New York: Hyperion, 1996: 9-20.

Callahan, Joan C. *Menopause: A Midlife Passage.* Bloomington, IN: Indiana University Press,1993.

hooks, bell. *Sisters of the Yam: Black Women and Self-Recovery.* Boston: South End Press, 1993.

Moyers, Bill and Joseph Campbell. *Power of Myths.* New York: Parabola Books, 1989.

Goldsby Grant, Gwendolyn, Ph.D. *Menopause: The Challenge of the Change.* New York: *Essence* Magazine, 1998: 90.

Barbach, Lonnie, Ph.D. *The Pause.* New York: Dutton/Plume, 2000.

Morgan, Joan. *When Chickenheads Come Home to Roost.* New York: Simon & Schuster, 1999: 87.

Chapter 11

Katzenback, Jon R. *Real Change Leaders.* New York: Time Books, 1995.

Jeffers, Susan, Ph.D. *Feel the Fear and Do It Anyway.* New York, Ballantine Books, 1988.

Bell, Chip R. *Managers as Mentors.* San Francisco: Berrett-Koehler, 1996.

Kotter, John P. *Leading Change.* Boston: Harvard Business School Press, 1996: 25.

Senge, Peter. *Fifth Discipline.* New York: Doubleday, 1994: 242.

Bagget, Byrd. *Dare to Soar.* Franklin, TN: Successories, Inc., 1996: 10-13.

Wright, H. Norman. *Winning Over Your Emotions.* Eugene, OR: Harvest House Publishers, 1998.

Hay, Louise. *You Can Heal Your Life.* Carlsbad, CA: Hay House, Inc., 1999: 18.

Mitioff, Ian. *Smart Thinking for Crazy Times.* San Francisco: Berrett-Koehler, 1998.

Moran, Beth. *Intuitive Healing.* Boston: Element Books, 1998: 16-17.

Giddings, Paula. *When and Where I Enter.* New York: William and Morrow & Company, Inc. 1984.

Clark Hine, Darlene, King, Wilma, and Linda Reed. *We Specialize in the Wholly Impossible.* Brooklyn, NY: Carlson Publishing, 1995.

Do Menopause with An Attitude Group Registration

Name of Group Leader:

Date of first meeting:

Themes:

Opening ritual:

Ongoing activities:

Discussion topics for first three meetings
1.
2.
3.

New topics to be addressed:

Celebration activities:

Send this registration to Carolyn Scott Brown at L.L. Brown International, Inc., 19435 68 Avenue South, Suite S105, Kent, WA, 98032 or email to llbrown@llbrowninc.com

Index

About the Author

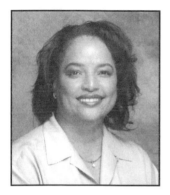

Carolyn Scott Brown is a psychologist, trainer, consultant, and life design coach. She teaches people how to transform their lives and reinvent their futures. Her Do Menopause with An Attitude seminars prepare women of color to celebrate the Second Half of Life.

Carolyn is president of L.L. Brown International, Inc., an educational corporation, where she develops motivational and educational programs for major corporations and non-profit organizations. After completing her master's degree in psychology at Columbia University, she worked in crisis intervention centers in New York City and was the Assistant Director of Student Affairs at Columbia University Business School. In 1982, she started her own consulting company. She inspires African-American women to see menopause as a gateway to a new future. Carolyn is a member of Delta Sigma Theta and lives in Seattle, Washington.

Barbara S. Levy is an internationally known women's health physician. She is acting as the medical consultant to L.L. Brown International, Inc. She lives in Federal Way, Washington.